Don't Let "IT" Get You!

Don't Let "IT" Get You!

An Empowering Health and Fitness Guide for Women

Joy Ohayia

iUniverse, Inc.

New York Lincoln Shanghai

Don't Let "IT" Get You!
An Empowering Health and Fitness Guide for Women

iUniverse books may be ordered through booksellers or by contacting:

iUniverse
2021 Pine Lake Road, Suite 100
Lincoln, NE 68512
www.iuniverse.com
1-800-Authors (1-800-288-4677)

Because of the dynamic nature of the Internet, any Web addresses or links contained in this book may have changed since publication and may no longer be valid.

ISBN: 978-0-595-46709-9 (pbk)
ISBN: 978-0-595-91005-2 (ebk)

Printed in the United States of America

I dedicate this book to all of the women I know and to all of the women I hope to meet in the future.

Many Blessings and Stay Healthy!

Acknowledgments

"I can do all things through Christ who strengthens ME. Phil 4:13"

To my Lord and Savior Jesus Christ, Thank you!

To: My Mother, Ruby
My Father's Spirit, Willie "Floyd"
My Husband, Chiji
My Sons Chikezie and Kemji
My Brother, Nate
My family and friends
I love you, thank you for your support.

To Tiffany Reed of TR Publishing Group, Inc, without you this book
would still be a dream.

45 Quest Lane

It's Saturday, 6 a.m.
She slips out of bed
Her sleeping husband
Lifts his head
Then buries it
Underneath a pillow
Quietly
She heads to the bathroom
Washes her face
Noticing the mirror
Imitating her gaze
She frowns at her sleepy eyes
Staring
Searching to find
The confidence inside
Refreshed and dressed
She grabs her shoes
Holding them as she ballets
Past her children's rooms
In the elements
She wonders
If she has lost her mind
Her weary eyes straining to see
Through the sunlight
It's time
Her time
Her body
Her race
She's off
Holding a steady pace
Sweat slowly starts to
Decorate her face
She starts to tire
But presses on
She turns the curb
Her sight set on the goal
An outpour of achievement
Cleanses her soul
Back where she started
She bends to catch her breath
Rising
She lifts her hands to the sky
Her eyes wide
She won!
She won!
She beat "IT"!

By: Tiffany "TRuth" Reed

CONTENTS

Introduction

I hated my corporate job but I loved the check!

I left early the day before "IT" happened. That same day a co-worker called me and said, "Are you okay, where are you? They laid three people off today, there's supposed to be four."

The following day I dressed very casual, I remember I had a 9'oclock meeting that morning. I noticed that while I was speaking, my manager refused to make eye contact or take note of anything I said. On my way out of the meeting a colleague who usually ignored me said, "Take care". Then my manager said, "Joy I need to speak with you".

I walked out of the conference room and never walked back in. I sat down and he said, "Your job has been terminated".

I said, "Okay good, how long will this take? I want to move my nail appointment up". As I left the building some of my colleagues looked sad, some even cried, I was thinking *Don't cry for me Argentina, this is great, I'm out of bondage!*

Two weeks later my dream was born.

Everyone advised me to use my newfound freedom to discover my passion. The answer hands-down, toes crossed was health and fitness. I have always been an athlete, I earned four individual records for sprinting and after over 20 years, two remain untouched. My first thought was, I need a company name it has to be big and attainable, "QuantumQuest!" Soon after, I opened a fitness club for women located in Central New Jersey. It was September 30, 2005 to be exact. I will admit, I was nervous and the process was overwhelming. So much that I did not realize the club was mine, until my husband and I were walking through it and I said, "They have to change that."

My husband looked at me and said, "Who? *They* is you!"

Okay, so now you are probably wondering why you should continue to read my book. Well for starters, I am a certified member of the American Fitness Professionals and Associates (AFPA). I specialize in the areas of wellness, personal training and nutrition. I am a nationally ranked sprinter, with four individual records. After 20 years, two remain untouched. I have been the health and fitness listen-up expert for dazzlin-diva.com since January of 2007. That same year Insight Publishing selected me as one of 14 powerhouse professionals in a book series titled, *Blueprint for Success*. As a member of the National Speakers Association, I motivate others to live life to its fullest and healthiest extent. I am an alumna of Stony Brook University College of Engineering. I also have a Masters degree in applied math and statistics from Rutgers University. But, before all of that, I am a wife, mother, daughter and friend like you. I am happily married to a supportive husband, with two teenage sons that drive me nuts with their social schedules. I want you to know that maintaining a healthy lifestyle does not require diet pills, six hours a day or lots of money. I want you to know that I did it with a splash of passion, a sprinkle of determination and a spice called courage; with the same ingredients, you can too.

You would not believe the downpour of negativity I endured after the layoff. People asked me how I was going to pay my bills, they asked for copies of my resume, so they could help me find a job, some so-called friends even cut me off. Mind you, these people were supposed to be supportive networks, while I set out to fulfill a life long dream. I shudder to think of where I could be mentally, physically and emotionally if I allowed others to have power over me. I am not claiming to be perfect or indestructible. I honestly hope to speak to someone in these chapters, I hope my experiences and professional advice will influence your future health related decisions in a positive way.

"Getting into our BEST physical and mental shape is the investment WE make today for many healthy tomorrows."

Chapter 1: What are my "Its"?

What are "Its"? "Its" are competing priorities that hinder us from achieving the things we want in life. This chapter focuses on "Its" that block us from achieving a healthy lifestyle. The truth is, we all desire to be fit and healthy, but we find millions of reasons not to follow through. Everyone has "Its" including me. A huge "It" for me was my corporate job. I ran two to three miles every morning just to keep my sanity! Running was a huge stress reliever; it cleared my mind and prepared me for the office nonsense. Another "It" was pregnancy, I gained 65 pounds with my first child, lost the weight, and then put on another 70 pounds with my second child.

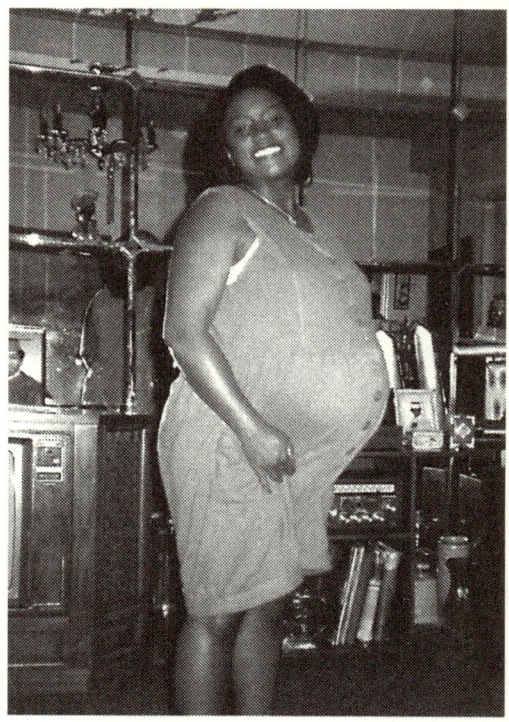

Here I am nine months pregnant with Kemji my second son.

I almost lost my kids, so the doctor told me to stay home. I couldn't move around so exercising was completely out of the question. The only thing I could do was eat and eat I did. During my pregnancy a friend asked, "What are you going to do with all of your clothes?"

I said, "You can borrow them, but I want them back."

Guess what, I got them back! Again, it came down to me. I knew what size I didn't want to be, so I made a lifestyle change. My doctor said I would never be small again. Guess I fooled him!

I hear "Its" all of the time; it does not matter where I am or what I am doing. If I am chatting on the phone with a friend, working with a client or speaking at an engagement "Its" always find a way to creep into the conversation. I duck periodically, because "It's" bounce off the walls at QuantumQuest too! The great news is that there are ways to defeat "Its", so you can achieve your healthy goals. Chart 1-1 displays some common "Its" and some strategies to defeat them.

Chart 1-1

Common "ITS"	Strategies around "ITS"
Time	Figure out what you are willing to give-up Keep a planner to manage your time
Self Induced Pressure	Remember who you are seeking to please … YOURSELF!
Family	Take care of you while they are occupied
Work	Use that stress in a positive way, sweat! I'll show you how
Money	Squats, Sit-ups, Running and Walking are free
Social Circles	Surround yourself with positive people, encouragement from like-minded people goes a long way

"Believe your determination and commitment is larger than ANY obstacle"

Time is the #1 "It", here is why, men *"take"* the time, women *"make"* the time. I have a friend who complains constantly about her growing dress size, but does nothing about it. Without blinking, she would swear she does not have time in a court of law. Her husband on the other hand is an aikido student and faithful member of Gold's gym for years. His work-out clothes include armor wear and a weight belt, which rest conveniently next to his golf clubs in the trunk of his car. This proves my point; he decided what he wanted to do then, designated the time to make it happen. What do we do? That's right, We think about everybody else. By the time, were finished fixing, listening and encouraging it's time for bed, so we can do it all over again! What would the average size of the American women be if we took time for ourselves? I bet my treadmill it would not be a size 14!

I know you want to be available to your children; I know you want to have dinner ready and trust me, I know you want to have energy for your husband and you will. Once you decide to take care of yourself first, I guarantee you will notice a surge in your energy and productivity at home and at work. Taking care of you makes you mentally, physically and emotionally ready to take care of everyone else without feeling resentful. I did it, here's how. I realized I could give up my lunch break. Instead of going out with my colleagues to listen to the office gossip, wasting gas and money; I utilized the company's gym for 30 to 45 minutes, then I showered and ate a salad drizzled lightly with balsamic vinaigrette at my desk. My point is that there is always time, we just have to be like our male counterparts and *"take"* it. If you are a stay at home mom finding the time to workout after taking care of the little ones is no easy task. Here is a suggestion. Have you noticed how devoted you are to watching your favorite shows? No matter where you are, you can look at the sun's position and instantly remember your soap, well, you can do the same for your workout. Ever thought about exercising while watching the show, I bet you would not realize the burn in the middle of a sit-up, because you'd want to lift up as quickly as you could to see what General Hospital's Sonny was going to do next!

Self-induced pressure is another common "It". When we decide to better ourselves, it gets overwhelming. It feels like everybody is watching and sometimes secretly hoping you fail, I experienced this first hand in my own home. Two weeks before the club opened my husband received his PhD, so I threw a congratulatory party for him. Sometime after, I learned that during the party a mutual friend of ours whispered, "She's going to fail" to another guest. This man like most of our friends assumed two things one, that I was going back into corporate America and two that my sons would have to leave private school. They were wrong. No matter what anybody said, I had to do what was right for me and so do you. Do not let negative people stop you from being happy or healthy. I cannot explain the completion I feel within myself, all because I did something for me in spite of what folks thought or said.

Another popular "It" is the family, in the introduction, I mentioned how incredibly, active my boys are; some moms might see this as an inconvenience, but I see it as free time. I work out, while they are at practice, hanging out with friends or studying with a tutor. This way I know they are safe and occupied while I take care of me. Honestly, I think I wrote half of this book in the bleachers at track meets!

When my boys were young, I had to find creative ways to exercise without leaving my husband for a long period of time. One solution was the "lunch break workout" the other took place on the weekends. I would wake up at about 5 am while my family was asleep to run at a local track, this way my husband only had to be around once the boys woke up. My husband hated the fact that I ran so early protected by nothing but reflectors, so he bought me a treadmill. I must admit I was not ecstatic about the gift because I never liked them, but at the same time; I was complaining of knee pain. Pavement was the causing factor. I did not know that pavement was rough on the knees; being a nationally ranked sprinter, I could not have that, so I gave in and now I love my treadmill. The treadmill is a compromise, because I get to workout whenever my heart pleases and my family knows exactly where I am. An important thing for us as women to remember is that our health and well-being are just as important as doing the laundry, grocery shopping and checking homework. Now raise your hand if you think you are the only one that can do the household chores right! The key to managing it all is to humble yourself enough to accept help when it is offered. If no one offers, delegate. Just try it to lift some of the burden off your shoulders.

Another discouraging "It" is work. A great way to make a positive life-style change at work is to include your co-workers. I had a salad entourage … seriously. The café would automatically start making salads as soon as they saw us coming down the stairs. Some co-workers would report their lunchtime choices to me! The key to allowing your healthy lifestyle to flourish at work is to stay secure, do not let office politics influence you, sure it is tempting to patronize a restaurant for a glass of wine, stuffed shells or a classic cheeseburger and fries but is it worth your life's longevity, no. Not to mention the money you'll save.

"Me. My satisfaction, health and happiness start with me."

Money, this "It" is another top excuse for why we neglect ourselves. A membership at a local gym can start as low as $30 a month, still I find myself constantly convincing women to invest in themselves. A common excuse is "I don't think my husband will approve." That is my cue to explain that, one of my personal long-term goals is independence. If my husband has to take care of me for more than four days, I get mean, so it is a problem for both of us! From my perspective, this dedication to health and fitness is a nest egg for happy and healthy retirement years. This usu-ally gives the unsure something to think about on the drive home. I am happy to announce that they usually return within a few days with a deposit.

When dealing with money it is important to get your priorities in order. For example, we usually treat ourselves to manicures, pedicures or appointments at the beauty shop twice a month. Which is great, these things do wonders for our self-esteem. My goal is to bring attention to the time and money spent in these establishments. Think about it, we spend at least two hours in the nail salon. After we pay for the manicure, pedicure and eyebrow wax, it cost at least $40. Let's not even discuss how long we are in the hair salon (that can be an all day event) with all of the coloring, treatments, extensions and the hour nap under the dryer it can cost well over $80.

So, by now, you are thinking, ok Joy what are you saying? I'm saying you only need 30 minutes at least three times a week to exercise and it doesn't have to cost anywhere near what you spend on a beauty day.

Peer pressure is alive and well! That is why Social circles are "Its". Remember the gossip from high school hallways, well surprise, surprise, it has found a platform in every social facet of our lives; believe it or not, we like celebrities have paparazzi too. Think about it, if you hire a gardener, buy a car or change your drapes the entire neighborhood knows about it. Once they figure out your schedule and notice your workout gear, you will have a problem. When you become determined to move forward people will try to discourage you. For example, let's say you are wearing your favorite t-shirt, sweats and sneakers armed with a water bottle and a towel, heading to the car when suddenly you hear "Look at her, who does she think she is? She isn't going to lose that weight!" You may be tempted to respond in a not so "lady-like" way. Instead, smile, wave and hit the gym using the jealousy as motivation instead. Besides, nothing says mind your business like shopping bags full of clothes two sizes smaller! On the other hand, you can try to incorporate the paparazzi into your fitness plan using the buddy system. I must admit I am not a big fan of the buddy system, because people are not reliable. I tried the buddy system and it worked well for six months, but eventually my buddy abandoned me because of "It" number 4: work! That could have discouraged me but I had already decided to run with or without her. I was fully committed to keeping my sanity.

Stress is another "It" that hinders us from performing at our best. We declare peace with ourselves everyday, but then the phone rings, the special man in our life does "it" again, our kids' start working our very last nerve, and to top it off, the bills show up in pink envelopes, not in support of breast cancer research; but because they are past due. What do we do? Stress! We become miserable, irritable, sensitive and all together fed up!

When it comes to stress like Nike, we just do it. Stress is a universal occurrence that affects everyone with a pulse. It affects us physically, mentally, socially and emotionally. While, we all face the same trials and tribulations, our bodies react differently when attacked by stress. The chart below displays the four categories of stress and common symptoms.

Chart 2-2

Physical	Mental	Social	Emotional
Headaches	Confusion	Isolation	Depression
Backaches	Inability to con-centrate	Sudden Out-bursts	Anxiety
Insomnia	Forgetfulness	Reduced Sex Drive	Self-Doubt
Tension in Muscles	Fatigue	Loneliness	Frustration

Stress usually arises in response to our body's sudden demand for action or change. Some examples of stress prone situations are funerals, college exams, family drama, money troubles, pregnancy, busy schedules, illness, the workplace, buying a home/car, weddings and the list goes on.

We cannot avoid stress, but here are some tips to help reduce the amount of stress in our lives.

STRESS-LESS Tips

Chart 3-3

LOVE YOURSELF	Say NO without feeling guilty You are not superwoman

<u>Chart 3-3</u> (Continued)

<u>ORGANIZE</u>	**Use a daily planner to prioritize your tasks** **This will give you a sense of control and reduce anxiety**
<u>EXERCISE</u>	**Yes, I said the E word! Walking/Running is great for relieving stress, grab an IPod and get moving!**
<u>TREAT YOURSELF</u>	**Relax: Schedule massages, bubble baths and movie nights**
<u>GO to BED</u>	**Small problems seem gigantic when you're tired, so get some rest**
<u>Chew and Sip Properly</u>	**Less bread, grease and cheese** **More fruit, water and tea**
<u>FORGIVE</u>	**Carrying a grudge requires too much energy and keeps you in bondage, free yourself**

Take this time to write down any additional "Its" in your life.

_____

_____

_____

_____

_____

_____

_____

_____

_____

_____

_____

_____

_____

_____

_____

_____

Now turn those "Its" into a motivational list. For each "It" write two ways you can overcome them.

_____

_____

_____

_____

"No matter the direction of the wind, I'm moving forward."

Chapter 2: Defining the Beauty that is Me

There are three common body types: ectomorph, mesomorph and endomorph. The purpose of this chapter is to evaluate your *current* shape to identify your body type. In learning this, we are able to understand our bodies; including why we gain weight in certain areas, why we sometimes experience difficulty gaining muscle/weight and how to split our time between cardio and muscle toning to gain the results we desire. Before we go any further, understand that no body type is greater than the other each type is equally exquisite. I say that because you cannot change your body type. Your bone structure will not allow such a change. For example, if you are an endomorph, you cannot become an ectomorph or if you are an ectomorph, you cannot become a mesomorph. Since, we are *born* into a body type, our goal, is to *accept* our body in its *current* state, then move on to make it a healthy equally toned masterpiece.

Are you an Ectomorph?

Ectomorphs are slim body types that are linear in shape with narrow hips, short upper bodies, and long arms and legs. If this is your body type, people have brought attention to the fact that your muscle and bone structures are visible and you have less fat and muscle mass than most people. Well now, you can stick your "bony" chest out and tell them you belong to an exclusive, yet small percentage of the population. Your body type is common among basketball players and supermodels, yes supermodels so work it! Being an ectomorph has its advantages. A great advantage is a fast metabolism, meaning you burn calories even while resting. You also have a high aerobic endurance, which is a sign of a strong cardiovascular system, which helps you to maintain that lean body. Some real life examples of ectomorphs are WNBA star Lisa Leslie and Supermodel Heidi Klum.

I know being the "skinny" one in the group isn't always easy. You have probably tried to gain weight and muscle definition ending in great disappointment. This challenge is common among ectomorphs. Another common obstacle for this body type is the fact that body your thin physique, which is made of small bones and joints, are especially vulnerable to injury during extracurricular activities. But don't get it twisted, being an ectomorph is not a bad thing, your petite muscles and joints are naturally flex-ible; this helps to prevent injuries as you progress in age. However, if you continue to experience difficulty putting on healthy weight and muscle, you should contact your doctor; this may be a sign of a dysfunctional thy-roid or diabetes.

A common myth among your body group is that you can eat anything and not gain an ounce—this is false—fat will build inside if you do not take care of your body. If muscle toning is not apart of your workout rou-tine, you risk gaining a higher fat to muscle ratio, which overtime comes to equal "not so lovely love handles". Remember being thin does not neces-sarily mean you are healthy. Without a nutritional diet and regular exer-cise, you risk future battles with high cholesterol, hypertension, and obesity. A beautiful exterior is your reward for a healthy interior.

Suggested Workout for Ectomorphs

A general goal for all ectomorphs should be to workout three to four times per week. Your workout should include the three components of fitness: cardiovascular activity, muscle toning and stretching. This combination is essential to any balanced workout. You can mix and match your workout, however you choose. For example, if you exercise two to three days a week, it is best to combine your cardio and muscle toning workouts. If you have four or more days set aside, you can alternate activities, like cardio on two days and muscle toning the other two days.

Muscle strength and conditioning = 60% of your total workout time
= Time Well Spent
Cardiovascular activity   = 40% of your total workout time

Your main goal is to increase muscle mass. Try to spend the larger per-centage of your exercise time doing muscle toning exercises, but do not, I repeat do not forget to condition your heart, after all it is the hardest work-ing muscle in your body. You can accomplish this by walking, biking, run-ning, rollerblading or swimming.

Are you a Mesomorph?

A mesomorph is the muscular body type. Their shape is rectangular with thick bones and muscles coupled with tight and well-defined abdominals, thighs, buttocks and calves. Their hips are the same width of their shoulders. If this is, your body type "gym rats" envy your ability to gain muscle easily. Don't apologize! Mesomorphs just happen to be naturally athletic looking individuals full of energy and extremely competitive. Olympic gymnast Carly Patterson and Tennis star Serena Williams are good examples of this body type. Yes, you have it going on, but like all body types, if a proper diet and consistent exercise are not routine you are at risk for obesity. Your "heavenly" body can and will fall to the wayside, if it becomes sedentary and burdened with a high-fat and/or high calorie diet. The greatest health threat to mesomorphs is cardiovascular disease, prevented through various healthy activities such as walking, running, rollerblading, bike riding and swimming.

I previously mentioned your unique ability to gain muscle easily, this is highly beneficial in the exciting journey of achieving a healthy body weight. As your body mass increases so does your metabolism. A speedy metabolism and strong muscles help to support and protect your skeletal frame. This is crucial, since our bones naturally decrease in density, as we age.

While mesomorphs have a lot going for them, there are some challenges. This body type gains fat as easily as muscle. If this is a growing issue for you, it is imperative that you increase your cardiovascular workouts to combat the fat. Another challenge to being a mesomorph is that at times you appear to look heavier than what you actually are due to your thick bones and muscles, which tighten on occasion, this can be controlled by consistent stretching especially before and after a workout.

If you are thinking this body type sounds familiar, but you do not meet all of the criteria, relax, there is nothing wrong with your DNA! The mesomorph body type has two sub groups.

1. Meso-Ecto: As a meso-ecto, you generally have a smaller bone frame, but resemble the muscle size and build of mesomorphs. Meso-ectos also have a tendency to be lean, similar to the ecto-morph, yet their natural strength is greater than that of the ecto-morph.

    This is my body type. I have excelled in track and field, a sport that requires great strength, short bursts of energy, and lots of power. I am a Nationally Ranked Collegiate and Masters Sprinter in the 55M and 100M events. Track is my passion, I eat, breathe and sleep track. My workout regime includes running 3.4 miles per day for five days, resistance training on two days and abdominal work for five days. My workout incorporates the three components: warm up (cardio), stretching (flexibility), resistance training (depends on the day of the week), core/abdominal exercises, cool down (cardio), and final stretch (flexibility).

2. Meso-Endo: As a meso-endo, you have the ability to retain a great deal of muscle mass. However being a meso-endo also makes you vulnerable to extra unevenly distributed fat. Meso-endos can usually combat the extra fat by allotting days and times for cardio exercises to stabilize a healthy body weight.

Suggested Workout for Mesomorphs

Here is a general recommendation: set a goal to work out three to four times a week. Your workouts should include cardiovascular activity, muscle toning, and stretching and can be broken down into half hour increments each day or you may opt to combine your cardio and toning exercises within the same day. Here is an example: if you choose to work-out three days (never consecutively) combine your cardio and toning exercises on all three days, however if you can add more days, try alternating your activities from day to day. Since you tend to put on muscle easily, you may not need to do a conditioning workout more than once or twice a week.

Be aware that muscle soreness the next day or two is normal, since muscle fibers break during exercise then, increase in size as they mend. If you over train, your body will give you warning signs such as a decrease in your ability to perform, sudden flu or cold and/or cold sores on your lips. I know that I am not a physician; however, these symptoms are usually signs of a weakened immune system. This can occur from inadequate rest intervals in between workouts. To avoid this do not train the same muscle group two days in a row.

*Tip: Give each muscle group at least two days of rest between workouts.

Muscle strength and conditioning = 40% of your total workout time
=Time Well Spent
Cardiovascular activity   = 60% of your total workout time

To maintain a healthy body fat percentage, working out aerobically four to five times per week is best. Here is an example of a general routine: if you exercise five days a week, 60% of the time you should cross train (bike, run, spin or swim) for your cardio workouts, spend the remaining 40% on muscle toning exercises.

Meso-ecto Workout:
Muscle strength and conditioning = 50% of your total workout time
= Time Well Spent
Cardiovascular activity   = 50% of your total workout time

Here is an example—if your schedule allows you to workout for one hour three days a week (Monday, Wednesday, Friday), you need to balance your routine, so that you do equal amounts of cardio and muscle toning exercises.

Workout Meso-endo:

Muscle strength and conditioning = 40% of your total workout time
                                      = Time Well Spent
Cardiovascular activity   = 60% of your total workout time

It is wise to focus on cardiovascular exercises. Set a goal for yourself to workout four to five times per week doing cardio endurance training and then incorporate muscle—conditioning exercises one to two days a week.

"It's none of my business what people say or think about me."—Anonymous

Are you an Endomorph?

If you are an endomorph, you have a curvaceous body! As an endomorph, your body fat settles into the lower regions of your body, predominately your lower abdomen, hips, and thighs, rather than evenly throughout the body. This body type resembles an hourglass. When an hourglass is turned upside down the sand settles at the bottom. The endomorph body type acts the same way. This body type has small to medium bones, limbs that are shorter in relation to the torso and musculature that is not well defined. While all body types are prone to excessive weight gain, the endomorph faces a higher inclination towards obesity. Some real life examples of this body type are R&B singer and Actress Beyonce Knowles and my favorite talk show host Oprah Winfrey.

The American Heart Association says abdominal fat deposition is more hazardous than the fat in the butt and leg area, because it is stored closer to the heart forcing it to work harder. This fat increases the danger of heart disease, diabetes, stroke, some cancers, and high blood pressure. The perfect combination: consisting of the proper nutrition intake and consistent exercise can prevent these illnesses. I hope that aside from all of the "Its" in your life, your health is becoming your first concern. Maintaining a healthy body weight can reduce your risk for devastating diseases. No matter your age, or body type our ultimate goal is to achieve and maintain a healthy lifestyle. The first step is to make the perfect combination paramount!

Suggested Endomorph Workouts

This particular body type needs a little more attention. Therefore, your long—term goal should be to workout four or more times a week. The most important thing is to stay active with cardio, muscle toning, and stretching as the three standard parts of every workout session. Endurance training through cardio is important, because it helps us to maintain a healthy body fat percentage. Your voluptuous frame makes any type of high impact cardio activity hard to do it also puts excessive strain on your joints. Therefore, to lose that excess body fat, your workouts should consist of low impact cardio activities such as walking, swimming (swimming exercises every muscle in the body) and rollerblading.

Muscle strength and conditioning = 30% of your total workout time
                                      =Time Well Spent
Cardiovascular activity   = 70% of your total workout time

You should also add muscle-toning exercises to your workout program for at least three days a week. Here is a secret, focus on developing muscle proportionately. If you gain weight in your lower half, but your arms and upper body are thin, you should concentrate on upper-body muscle toning. Cardio endurance and building muscle are your two key factors in developing a well-balanced physique inside and out.

The moment of acceptance has arrived.
Complete the following sentence.
I am a _____and proud of it!
            Insert Body Type

Now write down the areas of your body you would like to improve.

_____

_____

_____

_____

_____

_____

_____

_____

_____

_____

_____

Considering the suggested workout for your body type and the areas you wish to improve decide on a plan of action. Be as detailed as possible.

For Example: I will set aside 45 minutes and 3 days of each week to exercise.... Tuesday, Thursday and Saturday. As a mesomorph, I will focus on cardio and some weight training focusing on my arms, stomach and legs. Plan for sudden changes; write a back up plan as well. Then sign the bottom, this is your promissory note to yourself.

_____

_____

Are You Ready for a Change?

Use the assessment below to find out.

Place a check next to the statements that best describe you.

Level 1—Not Ready

___Taking care of me is the last thing on my "to do" list

___I am willing to take my chances against my family's medical history

___My time is strictly devoted to others

___Maybe next year

___I am tired all of the time a healthy lifestyle change would take all of my energy

___My career is more important than my health

___Money is no object

___If I suddenly start to exercise my friends will think I'm a health freak!

Level 2—Unsure

___I think I can take care of myself

___I am still debating I do not have the best family history

___I am willing to take a little time but I will not make any promises

___I want to live a healthy *closet* lifestyle

___Exercising and eating properly could increase my energy

___Job performance and health are equally important to me

___Money does not grow on trees but this time I am spending for me

___I know I should do this, but change is scary!

Level 3—Ready

___Now is the time to take care of me

___The family's medical history will not record me

___I will dedicate time to work on me

___ I don't care what people think, when can I start?

___ I am excited about a healthy change

___ If I'm healthy, I can perform better at work and home

___Money, I'm worth it, it won't go to waste

____A new lifestyle brings new experiences and new friends let's go!

The level with the most checks is your level of readiness.

What level are you? _____

"I am the star of my life."

If most of your checks are in **Level 1,** I understand, but I don't believe you. You are ready for some kind of change even if it is a small one because you are reading this book. Take a moment to congratulate yourself; you have just completed the first step to a lifestyle change by taking time for yourself. Close your eyes. Imagine yourself in your favorite outfit and guess what, you are not holding your stomach in! This vision is attainable if you let go of a few things that love to cling to your hips, thighs and buttocks. If you are interested and I know you are, I will show you how to eat and exercise in ways that are beneficial to your particular body type. Trust me I know lifestyle changes do not occur overnight. Start with small changes monthly, then weekly and before you know it, you will make healthy choices instinctively everyday. For example, at breakfast instead of the usual cup of coffee try an exotic tea. For snacks, forget about the office snack machine opt for your favorite fruit or nuts in moderation.

If most of your checks are at **Level 2,** I encourage you to choose a life of nutrition and activity. Think about your family's medical history; now imagine your health in five years, if you do not embrace a healthy lifestyle. If you are honest with yourself, there is a lot of uncertainty. Martha Stewart went to jail for good advice, let me help you with no sentence attached. I have a hot tip on health and wellness. These stocks have a solid reputation in disease prevention and longevity of ones life and guess what? The stock is free, but the results are priceless. Still not convinced, think about obstacles you have faced in the past. Remember how devastating those issues seemed, yet somehow you turned disappointment into a success. I am offering you the opportunity to make everyday a success simply, because you decided to do something for you.

If most of your checks are at **Level 3,** YOU GO GIRL! That is FAN-TASTIC, take a bow!

Before we move on let's recap, what we've learned so far. We have iden-tified our "Its", ways to avoid them, discovered our body type and assessed ourselves for readiness. We are ready for Chapter 3.

"It is time to take my own advice."

Chapter 3: I'm Ready for my Close-Up!

Tip—Always check with your physician before starting any fitness routine, especially if you have heart or respiratory concerns.

Now that you understand your body type, it is time to design a program just for you.

- First, we will evaluate your fitness level

- Then, create a chart to record your results

- Next, we will determine your goals

- Lastly, we will choose exercises to create your personalized program

Sounds like fun, let's get started!

Most people, (not you of course) love to talk about their strengths, but shy away from discussing their weaknesses. I have come to tell you that there is absolutely no reason to be ashamed of your limitations. We should embrace them by first, understanding what they are, then, use them as personal motivators. Let's face it, many people skip annual doctors visits and guard their actual clothing size like its' their pin number! "Keeping it real", I don't pay attention to the number sewn on the label; my main focus is how I feel in the clothes. If you are still playing "dress up" pretending you have the perfect body and a clean bill of health for years and years to come, now is the time to evaluate your current fitness level and make the life changing decision to be honest with yourself.

The first step in this process is to document your current body measurements in the Motivation & Fitness Evaluation chart provided. This chart is for your own personal enjoyment and motivation, because it helps you to get an idea of what your present fitness level is; it also allows you to track your progress during your workout program. *FYI*: I do not expect, nor would I ask you to carry this chart around at all times.

Another option, if you desire a precise measurement is to contact a professional for an evaluation. Physicians, health clubs, health and fitness fairs, health or therapy clinics, and YMCA's all provide fitness evaluations.

Grab a mirror, look at yourself and declare, "I am Beautiful!"

Now let's begin to measure objectively and effectively:

Motivation & Fitness Evaluation Worksheet

Start Date: _____

Measurement	Starting Measure	6 Week Measure	12 Week Measure	24 Week Measure
1-Resting Heart Rate				
2-Target Heart Rate				
3-Working Heart Rate				
4-Total Body Weight				
5-Dress Size				
6-Pant Size				
7-Shirt Size				
Body Fat Test:				
8-Chest				
9-Abdomen				
10-Triceps				
11-Thigh				

Muscular Strength & Endurance:				
12-Push-ups				
13-Curl-ups				
Flexibility:				
14-Ceiling Stretch				
15-Cardiovascular Test				
Measurements:				
16-Chest				
17-Arm				
18-Waist				
19-Hip				
20-Thigh				
21-Calf				

You will need the following items to complete this chart: a clock or watch, calculator, stop—watch, measuring tape and of course, basic workout gear: sports bra, t-shirt, and sweatpants. You don't want to wear anything constricting like jeans, because you want your skin to breathe. Last, but not least, you need sneakers with supportive innersoles. I personally recommend Spenco; they help to prevent shin splints and knee pain better than the innersoles sold in most sneakers. Their innersoles provide better cushioning for your feet, while they endure the added pressure during your cardio workouts. You can contact Spenco directly at 1-800-877-3626 or www.spenco.com

Tip: You should change your sneakers and innersoles every 9 months. If you walk/run more than 20 miles per week on a consistent basis (Hey you never know, you may develop a fancy for long cardio workouts!) You should replace your sneakers and innersoles every 6 months.

Below is the step-by-step process on how to complete this chart.

1—Resting Heart Rate

To get an accurate rate it best to check it as soon as you wake up, so after you give a groggy good morning to hubby, grab your wrist and start counting.

Here's how: Find your pulse, using the radial artery in your wrist or the carotid artery in your neck.

Tip: Do not use your thumb because it has a light pulse and can cause confusion while counting beats.

Once you find your pulse, you need to count the number of beats that occur within a 60-second period. *Short cut:* count the number of beats for 30 seconds then multiply that number by 2 this will also give you a 60 second count.

For example, if you count 35 beats in 30 seconds: 35 x 2 = 70 beats per minute.

2—Target Heart Rate

Your target heart rate gives you the high and low of your working heart rate range. The American College of Sports Medicine says it is best to maintain 55% to 90% of your maximum heart rate (MHR) while working out.

How to find the MHR: Use this formula, 220 minus your age = Your Maximum Heart Rate

For example, I am 45 years old. 220 - 45 = 175, 175 is my maximum heart rate.

Now let's find the target heart rate (THR).
Multiply your MHR with the low and high zone percentages
Low: 55% High: 90%

For example using my MHR,
175 (MHR) x .55 = 96.25, the low end of my THR.

175 (MHR) x .90 = 157.50, the high end of my THR.

*Don't forget to add these numbers to your chart.

3—Working Heart Rate

You calculate the working heart rate the same way you calculate the resting heart rate.
(By finding your pulse and counting your beats per minute.) The only difference is that you measure your heart rate while you are working out! So grab your sneakers and sweats and get moving! Run in place, dance, jump rope, power walk, jog etc.

Here's how: Get your legs moving for 10 to 15 minutes. After you feel like you are working at a good pace (a little sweat on the brow), stop, grab your watch, find your pulse, and start counting.

For example: To calculate this I might hop on the treadmill or jog outside for about 15 minutes then, stop to check my pulse. In 30 seconds, I usually count 75 beats.
Using the short cut, I multiply 75 by 2, which equals 150, 150 is my working heart rate.

I then calculate my THR:
[150 times .55 = 82.5]
[150 times .90 = 135]

According to the formula, I am working closer to the higher end of my THR, which is 157.50.

Target Heart Rate Training Zones

Age	50% Zone	70% Zone	Max. Rate
20 years	100	150	200
25 years	98	146	195
30 years	95	142	190
35 years	93	138	185
40 years	90	135	180
45 years	88	131	175
50 years	85	127	170
55 years	83	123	165
60 years	80	120	160
65 years	78	116	155
70 years	75	113	150

Short cut: To avoid the math you can purchase a heart rate monitor to strap around your chest or wrist. If you choose this option, I recommend Polar Electro Inc. Polar offers ten different models to choose from, you can contact them directly at 1-800-743-9248 or www.polarusa.com.

FYI: Spenco and PolarUSA are not paid advertisements. I recommend them based on my personal experience.

4—Total Body Weight

Do not be discouraged by the weight shown on the scale. The numbers can be very deceiving. For example, if you have a lot of muscle in your body, your body weight may seem a bit high. This is a good thing, because muscle weighs more than fat. A higher body weight sometimes indicates a healthy amount of muscle mass. On the other hand, if your weight is low there are two options to consider:

1. You are probably in great shape and have a balanced fat to muscle ratio, however, if you have not exercised in the last year this most likely is not the case.

2. Your low body weight may also indicate that you have a high body fat percentage and very little muscle. Always remember, fat does not weigh as much as muscle, so even though the numbers

on the scale are attractively low, you may not be healthy on the inside.

5, 6, 7—Dress, Pant, and Shirt Sizes

Different clothing manufacturers use different sizing scales, this explains why you're a 12 in some stores and an 8 in others. Therefore, to get accurate results write down the dress, pant, and shirt size that fits you best.

Tip: Make a note of the clothing manufacturer for each item.

8, 9, 10, 11—Body Fat Measurements

There are many ways to assess our body fat. However, for accurate results it is highly recommended that you ask a health professional to assist you. Testing fees range from free to over $100 with varying methods: calipers to water weighing. I also recommended that once you find a health professional you are comfortable with, you keep him/her for consistency and accuracy in your measurements.

You can compare your percentages with the average woman in the chart below:

Body Fat Percentages for Women

Age	20-30	30-40	40-50	50 +
Very Low Fat	to 17	to 18	to 20	to 21
Low Fat	17-20	14-17	20-23	17-21
Avg. Fat	21-23	18-21	24-27	21-24
Very High Fat	24-27	25-29	28-31	31-35
Excessive Fat	28 +	30 +	32 +	36 +

* 12% of fat is normal in physiological function of a woman's body.
*5% is normal for men.

Can I have 0% body fat?

It is impossible, even in cases of severe starvation, to have 0% body fat. Your body will not function properly without fat. Fat occurs in bone marrow, internal organs, brain and spinal cord. Women require more body fat for childbearing and other hormone-related functions.[1]

12—Push Ups

Push-ups are done on the toes or knees.

Here's how: get down on all fours, assume the standard hands and toes position or the bent knee position for less intensity, and back support. Now, push up until you are exhausted! Please don't give up after 2!

Push-Up Norms for Women[*]

Age	20-29	30-39	40-49	50-59	60 +
Excellent	49+	40+	25+	30+	20+
Good	34-48	25-39	20-34	15-29	5-19
Average	17-33	12-24	8-19	6-14	3-4
Fair	6-16	4-11	3-7	2-5	1-2
Low	0-5	0-3	0-2	0-1	0

[*] Family Education.com Workouts and Your Body 31 July 2007
<http://life.familyeducation.com/exercise/fitness/35975.html?page=4>

Don't forget to write down the number of push-ups you completed on your Motivation & Fitness Evaluation Worksheet.

13—Curl ups

Curl ups or abdominal curls are the best ways to tighten your abdominals and test your muscle endurance.

Here's how: Lie down on your back with your knees bent. (If needed have someone hold your feet to the floor.) Place your hands behind your head. Lift your chest to the ceiling and then lower yourself back down to the floor. Make sure you keep your chin off your chest. Remember to record your numbers. Repeat until exhausted.

---

1. Rhonda Gates Lifestyles by Rhonda Gates 2 June 2007
<http://www.rondagates.com/exercise/howfat.html>

Curl Up Norms[*]

	M (<35)	M (35-44)	M (45 +)	W (<35)	W (35-44)	W (45 +)
Excellent	60	50	40	50	40	30
Good	45	40	25	40	30	15
Marginal	30	25	15	25	15	10
Needs Work	15	10	5	10	6	4

[*] Topendsports.com Fitness Testing 26 July 2007
<http://www.topendsports.com/testing/tests/abendur.htm>

14—Stretch to the Ceiling

Your ability to extend your hamstrings is a good indicator of your spine, hip, and hamstring flexibility.

Grab something comfortable to lie on (not the couch!), a mirror or a partner to help determine your maximum stretch.

Here's how: Lie on your back with one leg lying on the floor. Raise the opposite leg up towards the ceiling by placing your hands behind your knee (for a better grip, interlock your fingertips). With your hands, pull your leg in towards your chest, keeping your knee as straight as possible and your foot flexed (your toes should be toward your nose). A measurement of good flexibility would be 80 or 90 degrees of hip flexion. What this means is that your leg will be perpendicular (at a right angle) to the floor.

Greater than 80 to 90 degrees of hip flexion = Excellent flexibility
Equal to 80 to 90 degrees of hip flexion = Good flexibility
Less than 80 degrees of hip flexion = Below average flexibility
Don't forget to record this on your worksheet.

15—Cardiovascular Test

The step test is an easy way to calculate your cardiovascular fitness.

Here's how: First locate your pulse, and then using a step or a sturdy box begin stepping up and down for 3 minutes. As soon as you are done, find your pulse and record the number of beats per minute on your worksheet.

Check your fitness level below:[2]

Fitness Level	Men (18-29)	Women (18-29)	Men (30-57)	Women (30-57)
Excellent	69-75	76-84	63-75	73-86
Good	76-83	85-94	77-90	87-100
Average	84-92	95-105	91-106	101-116
Fair	93-99	106-116	107-120	117-130
Poor	100-106	117-127	121-134	131-144

16, 17, 18, 19, 20, 21—Taking Measurements

You will need a measuring tape for this section.

Here's how: Measure the location points for each part of your body as described below:

16—Chest: Place the measuring tape along the nipple line.
17—Arm: The tape should cover the upper arm just below the armpit.
18—Waist: Find your most narrow point and measure.
19—Hips: Slide the tape up and down to find your widest point and measure.
20—Thighs: Find the widest point in your thigh (upper leg) and measure.
21—Calf: Search for the widest point and measure.

---

2. Topendsports.com Fitness Testing 26 July 2007
   <http://www.topendsports.com/testing/tests/abendur.htm>

Record your measurements on your Motivation & Fitness Evaluation Worksheet.

*Before you begin your exercise routine, please obtain clearance from your physician to continue. Discuss your plan and get an "ok" prior to starting a routine.

How conditioned are you?

Go back to you motivation worksheet and review your results for numbers 12, 13, 14, and 15. Compare to the norms provided for each measurement and determine your fitness category. If your scores fall into the excellent, good, and average range then you will move on to the Conditioned workout routine. If your scores fall in the fair, poor, marginal or below average range then you are in the Deconditioned workout routine.

If you ranked in the Deconditioned area, remember we need to begin somewhere. We will take it slow and build onto your routine. Do not be discouraged! Congratulate yourself on completing the assessment then, keep it moving.

Furthermore, besides, of your routine category the steps are the same, the only difference is in the number of sets and repetitions.

<u>Deconditioned Workout Routine</u>

Step 1: Select your Favorite Exercises

Select 1 to 2 exercises per muscle group. The following pages describe and show different exercises for various muscle groups, I recommend these exercises from my personal experience, but feel free to add some of your favorite exercises.

Step 2: Sets and Reps

Before we begin, we need to define the difference between a *set and repetition*. Repetition (rep for short) is the number of times you perform an exercise. The American College of Sports Medicine defines a set as a group of consecutive repetitions per weight training exercise reaching the maximum intensity for the entire set. Each set should contain between 8 to 10 reps.

For example:
Exercise: Bench Press
Repetitions (Reps): 8 to 10
Sets: 1 (for the first week of training)

When training my clients in the deconditioned workout routine, I start them all at one set. Then I move them on to two in some exercises and eventually all over the next 3 weeks. I found that progression works best with my clients. I like progression because it is also the safer approach, as opposed to jumping into a hardcore program from day one. My clients have not complained of any negative repercussions such as soreness or lack of desire to continue with the program. A progressive system increases the duration and level of intensity over time without overworking your muscles.

Step 3: How much weight should I use?

Progression is the key. You should start with light—weights and increase over time. Rule of thumb: If you can perform all of the reps for each set of a particular exercise, then increase the weight by a small amount. It is normal to experience muscle fatigue during the last few reps of your set. Fatigue is an indication that you are getting the most out of your workout.

Step 4: Cardiovascular Exercise

Cardiovascular health and fitness is defined as the ability of the heart to meet the demand of physical activities sustained for intervals of 20 minutes or more. In 2005, the U. S. Surgeon General issued a report recommending 30 minutes of moderate exercise per day. This may sound like a lot, but you can achieve 30 minutes in various ways such as walking to work, gardening, walking up stairs. I suggest that you focus on more intense activities such as walking briskly, jogging, or swimming. Focus on your target heart rate. If you reach your target, increase your duration. In doing this you increase your caloric expenditure and consequently see your desired results sooner! To warm up choose the cardio exercise you prefer and exercise for 5-10 minutes. If you are just starting a workout routine, I suggest a longer warm-up period. Here are some benefits of cardio activities:

Burn calories, body fat and maintain lean body mass
Improve your ability to exercise in hot weather
Decrease clinical symptoms of anxiety
Increase aerobic work capacity
Relieve stress and body tension
Reduce the risk of heart disease
Reduce the risk of some cancers
Decrease Resting Heart Rate
Decrease total cholesterol
Reduce blood pressure
Increase overall energy
Increase heart volume
Prevent Osteoporosis
Live longer!

It only takes 30 minutes of your day. Move your body and get your heart pumping! Move your arms and legs to reach your target heart rate. It's important to keep your heart in shape; it is the hardest working muscle in your body.

If your scores were in the excellent, good, and average range, then you will move on towards the **Conditioned workout routine**.

Step 1: Select your Favorite Exercises
Select 1 to 2 exercises per muscle group.

Step 2: Sets and Reps
Perform 3 sets (a group of consecutive reps) of each exercise you choose. Each set should contain 10 reps (the number of times you perform the exercise).

Example:
Exercise: Bench Press
Repetitions (Reps): 10
Sets: 3

Step 3: How much weight should I use?
Progression is the key. You should start with light—weights and increase over time. Rule of thumb: If you can perform all of the reps for each set of a particular exercise, then increase the weight by a small amount. It is normal to experience muscle fatigue during the last few reps of your set. Fatigue is an indication that you are getting the most out of your workout.

Step 4: Cardiovascular exercise
What is cardiovascular health? It is the ability of the heart to meet the demand of physical activities sustained for intervals of 20 minutes or more. In 2005, the U. S. Surgeon General issued a report recommending 30 minutes of moderate exercise per day. This may sound like a lot, but you can achieve 30 minutes in various ways such as walking to work, gardening, walking up stairs. I suggest that you focus on more intense activities such as walking briskly, jogging, or swimming. Focus on your target heart rate. If you reach your target, increase your duration. In doing this you increase your caloric expenditure and consequently see your desired results sooner! To warm up choose the cardio exercise you prefer and exercise for 5-10 minutes. If you are just starting a workout routine, I suggest a longer warm-up period. Here are some benefits of cardio activities:

Burn calories, body fat and maintain lean body mass
Improve your ability to exercise in hot weather
Decrease clinical symptoms of anxiety
Reduce the risk of some cancers
Relieve stress and body tension
Reduce the risk of heart disease
Increase aerobic work capacity
Decrease Resting Heart Rate
Decrease total cholesterol
Increase overall energy
Reduce blood pressure
Increase heart volume
Prevent Osteoporosis
Live longer!

It only takes 30 minutes of your day. Move your body and get your heart pumping! Move your arms and legs to reach your target heart rate. It's important to keep your heart in shape; it is the hardest working muscle in your body.

To stay motivated change your routine every couple of weeks. Select different muscle-toning exercises and/or cardio exercises to best suit your needs (based on your body type), enjoyment, and schedule.

Before we go any further, we need to learn how to stretch!
I know, I know, you feel like you've done a million things today so, by now you feel pretty warmed up. Well I have news for you, stretching goes much further than a simple touch of your toes. To get you warmed up to the idea, here are five ways to improve your stretching technique.

Warm-up Warm up by walking gently pumping your arms, or do a favorite exercise at low intensity for five minutes.

Target Major Muscle Groups Focus on your calves, thighs, hips, lower back, neck and shoulders.

Hold Each Stretch It takes time to lengthen tissues safely. Hold your stretches for at least 30 seconds and up to 60 seconds for problem areas. Then repeat the stretch on the other side.

Do Not Bounce Bouncing while stretching can cause small tears in the muscle. These tears leave scar tissue, which tightens the muscle.

Focus on Pain-Free Stretches Expect to feel tension while you are stretching. If this hurts, you have gone too far. Relax the stretch and try again.

If you have a chronic condition or injury, you may need to alter your approach to stretching. For example, if you have a strained muscle, stretching it regularly may cause further damage. To avoid this discuss the best ways to stretch with your doctor or physical therapist. If strenuous activity is completely out of the question at this time just stay active! Instead of parking in the closest space you can find, park further away and walk. Activities like gardening, outdoor activities with the kids, cleaning and painting can help you burn calories.

Stretching also has a number of benefits here are the top six.

Stretching—

1. **Increases Flexibility**—Flexible muscles can improve your daily performance. Tasks such as lifting packages, bending to tie your shoes or hurrying to catch a bus becomes easier and less tiring.

2. **Increases Range of Motion**—Good range of motion improves your balance, which will help keep you mobile and less prone to injury from falls, especially as you age.

3. **Improves Circulation**—Stretching increases blood flow to your muscles. Improved circulation can speed recovery after muscle injuries.

4. **Promotes Good Posture**—Frequent stretching keeps your muscles from getting tight, allowing you to maintain proper posture minimizing aches and pains.

5. **Relieves Stress**—Stretching relaxes the tense muscles that often accompany stress.

6. **Helps to Prevent Injury**—Preparing your muscles and joints for activity can protect you from injury, especially if your muscles or joints are tight.

As we enter the exercise portion of this program. Feel free to use the muscle-toning chart below to track your progress.

MUSCLE TONING CHART (Sample)

Begin Date: _____
(Write YOUR Goals here)

Date	Exercise	Weight	Reps	Sets	Notes
7/18	Chest Press	10 lbs	10	3	Felt good, increase weight
	Lunges with Weights	5 lbs	10	3	
	Bicep Curl	10 lbs	10	3	3rd set was challenging

Notes:

- Prior to beginning, any training consult your physician.
- Adequate warm-up and stretching exercises are recommended prior to resistance training/muscle toning, to loosen the muscles and prevent injury.

- Adequate cool-down and stretching exercises are recommended post resistance training/muscle toning, to prevent the stiffening of muscles.

Let's start with the upper body.

Push Ups

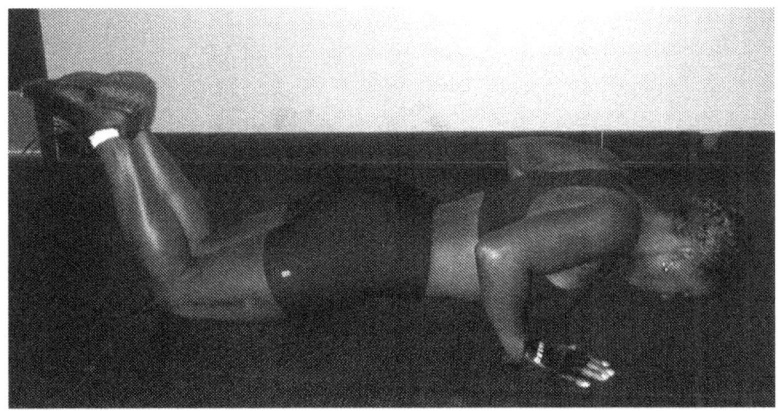

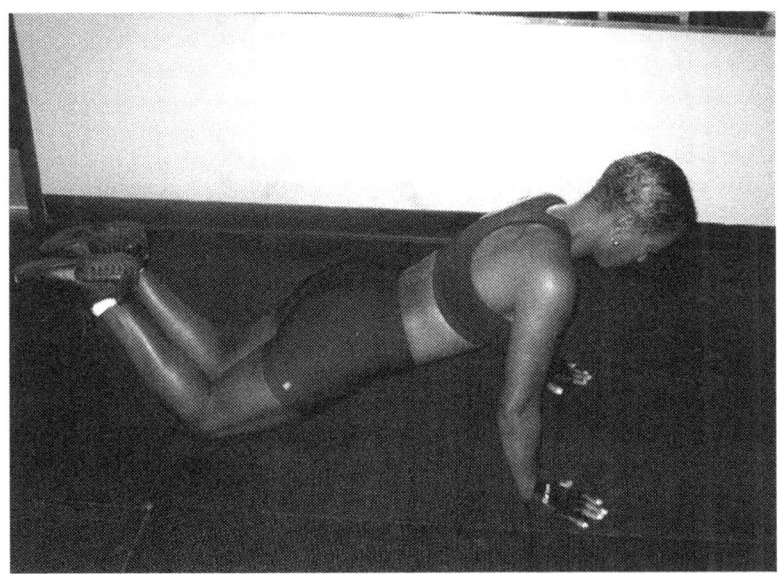

Be sure to perform push-ups on a mat or a carpeted floor for comfort. Breathing is KEY! It is important to exhale during the period of exertion (on your way up from the floor).

Steps:

1. Start on the floor with your hands and knees and place your hands slightly wider than shoulder width apart.

2. Slowly lower your chest towards the floor and push yourself back up.

3. Keep your back straight and head in alignment with your spine.

Deconditioned routine
Sets = 1
Reps = as many as you can
Increase your sets (maximum of 3 after 3 weeks)

Conditioned routine
Sets = 3
Reps = 10
Rest for 30 seconds in between sets

Target Areas: Pectorals, Biceps, Triceps (Chest and Arms)

Flys

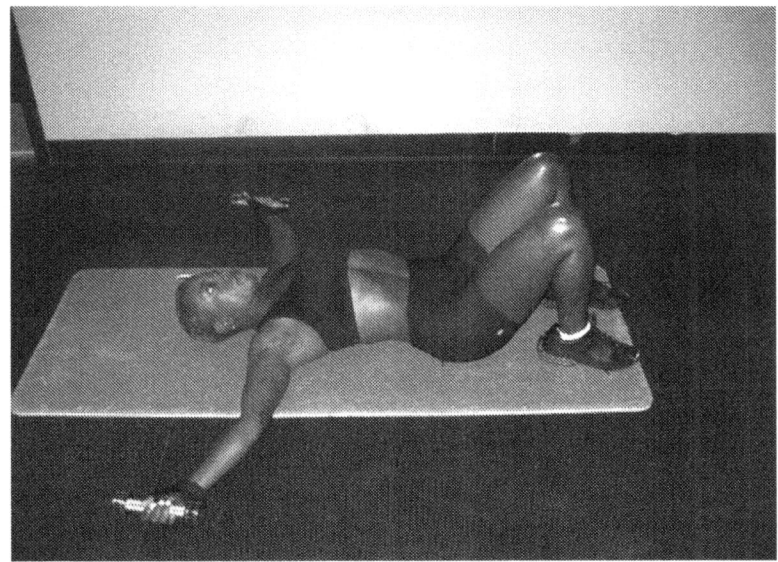

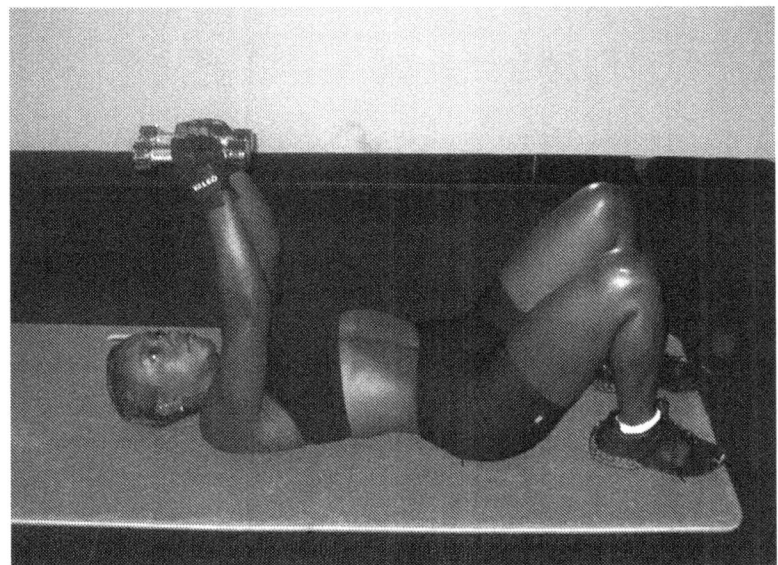

You will need weights for this exercise.

Contraindication (Warning) To prevent injury do not swing the weights.

Steps:

1. Lie on your back with your back flat and feet firmly on the floor.

2. With the dumbbells in your hands, extend your arms toward the ceiling with your palms facing in.

3. Slowly lower, your arms out to your sides back into the starting position.

4. Hold in your stomach to help build strength in your abs.

5. Always remember to breathe!

Deconditioned routine
Sets = 1
Reps = 8 to 10
Weights = 3 to 5 pounds
Increase your reps (maximum of 3 after 3 weeks).

Conditioned routine
Sets = 3
Reps = 10
Weights = 8 pounds or more
Rest for 30 seconds in between sets

Target Area: Pectorals (Chest)

Straight Arm Pull—Over

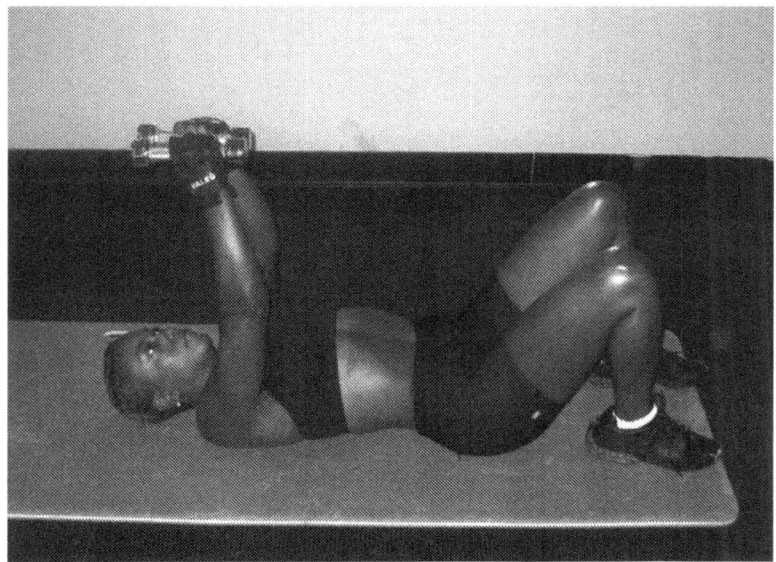

Be sure to hold the end of the dumbbell above the floor.

Steps:

1. Lie on your back with your feet firmly on the floor.

2. Hold one dumbbell in both hands and extend your arms over-head.

3. Slowly pull the dumbbell forward, stopping the movement over your chest.

4. Hold in your stomach to help build strength in your abs.

5. Exhale as you lift the dumbbell over your head.

Deconditioned routine
Sets = 1
Reps = 8 to 10
Weights = 3 to 5 pounds

Tips: If you are having difficulty completing this exercise, shorten your range of motion. Increase your reps (maximum of 3 after 3 weeks)

Conditioned routine
Sets = 3
Reps = 10
Weights = 8 pounds or more
Rest for 30 seconds in between sets

Target Areas: Pectorals (Chest)

Chair Dips

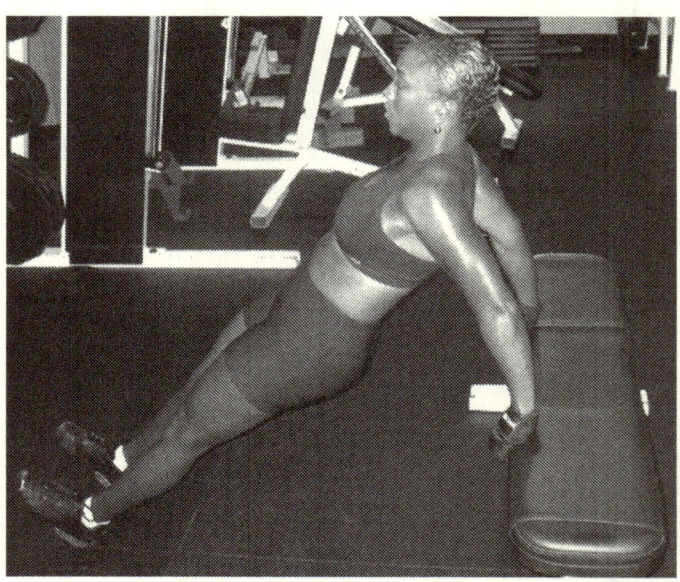

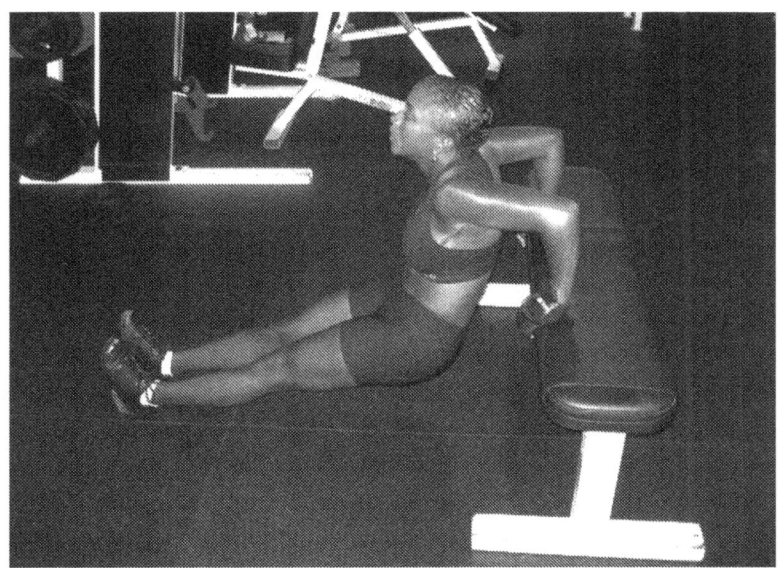

Chair dips are one of my favorite exercises; they target the muscles underneath the arm. All you need for this exercise is the edge of a chair (making it ideal for the office). If you feel uncomfortable during this exercise in the beginning that's normal, stick with it, you'll love the results. You will need a chair (without wheels) for this exercise.

Contraindications: Keep your elbows parallel to each other. Do not hyper-extend your wrists, keep them straight. For better results, move your body through the full range of motion.

Steps:

1. Stand in front of the chair, facing away from the chair's seat. As you sit down on the edge of the seat, place your hands behind your hips (also at the edge of the seat) and shoulder width apart.

2. Lift your butt off of the seat and walk your feet forward, your legs should be straight with toes pointed toward the ceiling. Slowly lower your body downward, being careful that your elbows do not bend to an angle smaller than 90 degrees.

3. Extend your arms, raising your body upward and supporting your weight with your arms.

4. Breathe!

5. Repeat.

Deconditioned routine
Sets = 1
Reps = 6 (or as many as you can)
Increase your sets (max 3 after 3 weeks)
*Do not be discouraged if you only complete one, slow progress is better than no progress.

Conditioned routine
Sets = 3
Reps = 10 to 12

Target Areas: Triceps

Hammer Curl

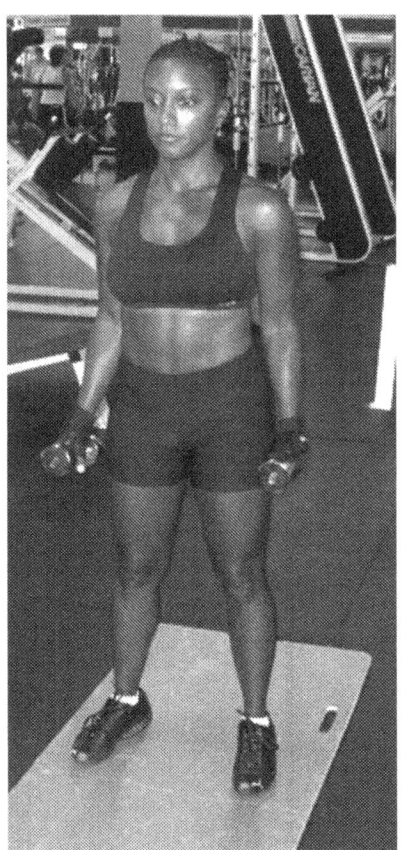 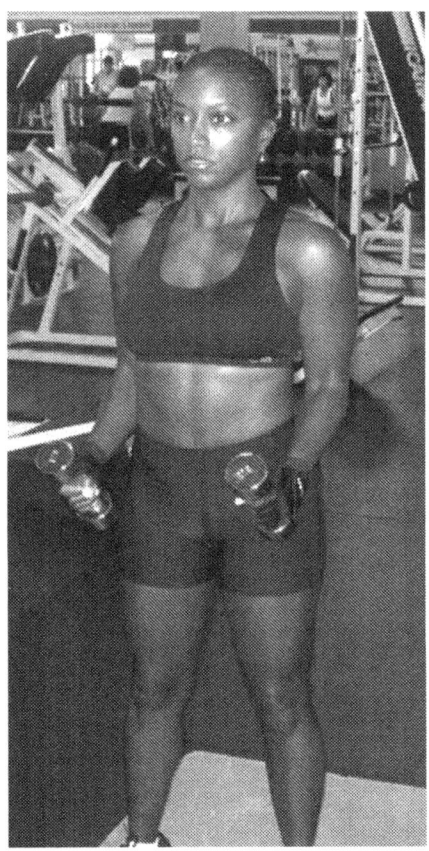

Add a dumbbell to firm, tone, and shape your arms.

Contraindication: To prevent injury do not swing the weights.

Steps:

1. Stand with your feet shoulder width apart and hold the dumbbells down by your sides.

2. Keeping your palms faced in toward your body slowly curl your hands up to your shoulders.

3. Concentrate on squeezing your biceps at the top of the range of motion and then release your arms to their starting position.

4. Hold in your stomach to help build strength in your abs.

5. Always Remember to breathe!

Deconditioned routine
Sets = 1
Reps = 8 to 10
Weights = 3 to 5 pounds
Increase sets and reps after 3 weeks.
Tip: Sit in a chair while you perform this exercise

Conditioned routine
Sets = 3
Reps = 10
Weights = 8 pounds or more
Rest for 30 seconds in between sets

Tip: Sit in a chair instead of standing.

Target Area: Biceps (Arms)

Alternate Curl

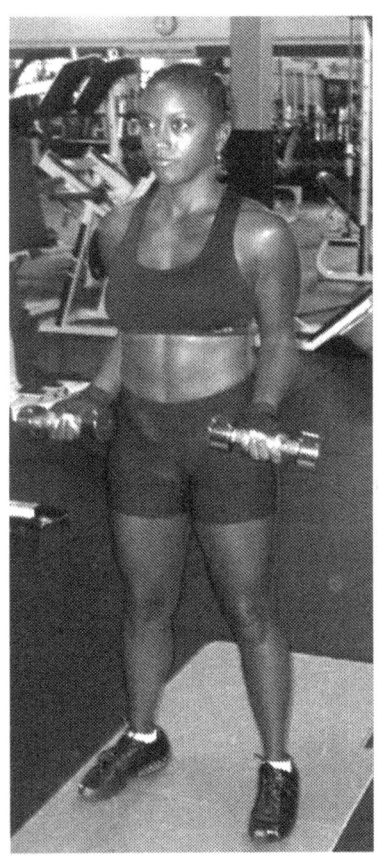
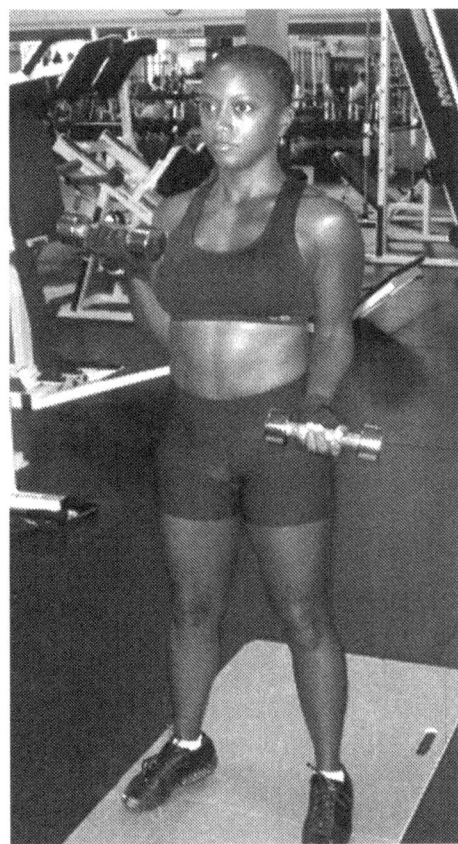

For maximum productivity, you will rest one bicep while working the other, allowing total concentration on the working bicep.

Contraindications: Do not swing weights.
Do not use your body's momentum to lift the weights and lastly, keep your torso still while lifting the weights.

Steps:

1. Stand with your feet and shoulder apart.

2. Hold your dumbbells by your sides with your palms facing away from your body.

3. Slowly lift one hand toward your shoulder, squeezing your biceps at the top.

4. Release your arm back to its starting position and repeat using the other arm.

5. Hold your stomach in and breathe.

Deconditioned routine
Sets = 1
Reps = 8 to 10
Weights = 3 to 5 pounds

Tip: Sit in a chair, the chair will provide support for your back.
Increase sets and reps after 3 weeks.

Conditioned routine
Sets = 3
Reps = 10
Weights = 8 pounds or more
Rest for 30 seconds in between sets

Target Areas: Biceps (Arms)

Overhead Extension

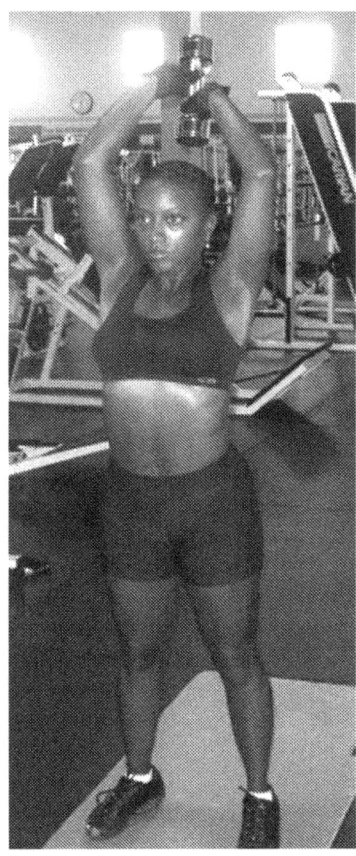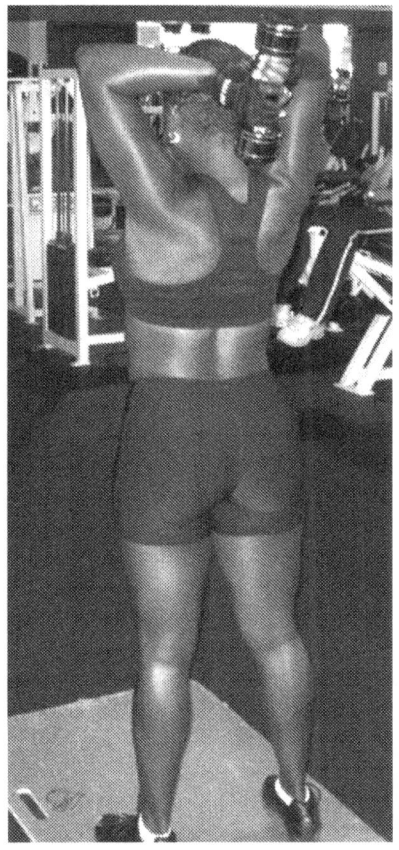

Use a chair or a stand. A chair helps to keep your back from swaying allowing you to focus your on your upper arms.

Contraindications: Be careful not to smack yourself with the weights!

Steps:

1. Stand with your feet together and knees slightly bent.
2. Hold dumbbell in both hands over your head.

3. Slowly lower the weight behind you.

4. Take the weight back to the starting position by extending your elbows and squeezing your triceps (back of upper arms).

5. Hold your stomach in to prevent arching in your back.

6. Breathe.

Deconditioned routine
Sets = 1
Reps = 8 to 10
Weights = 3 to 5 pounds
Increase sets and reps after 3 weeks.

Conditioned routine
Sets = 3
Reps = 10
Weights = 8 pounds or more
Rest for 30 seconds in between sets

Target Areas: Triceps (Arms)

Back lick

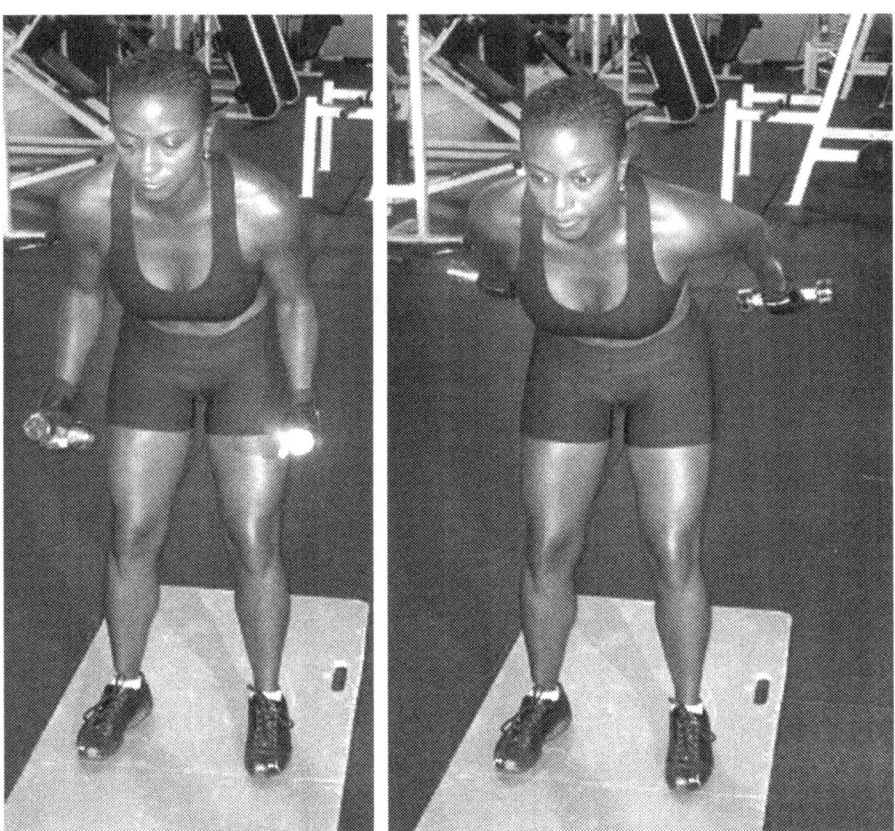

This exercise is spectacular in improving the condition of your triceps; they are located in the back of your upper arm.

Contraindications (Warning) Keep your back straight and head aligned with your spine. Keep your elbows to your sides so you can concentrate on your range of motion.

Steps:

1. Stand with your feet together and hold the dumbbells by your side.

2. Bend from the waist so your back is flat but with a slight arch.

3. Bring your elbows up so that the dumbbells are next to your side and your palms are facing the sides of your legs.

4. Slowly extend your elbows, pushing the weight behind you.

5. As you push the weight back, rotate your palms to the ceiling. As you return the weight to the starting position, rotate your palms back to the sides of your legs.

6. Squeeze your triceps at the top of the range of motion (the point where your elbows are fully extended) and release them to their starting position.

7. Hold in your stomach to support your back.

8. Breathe

Deconditioned routine
Sets = 1
Reps = 8 to 10
Weights = 3 to 5 pounds
Increase sets and reps after 3 weeks

Tip: If you experience back problems, sit in a chair and lean forward with your chest toward your knees.

Conditioned routine
Sets = 3
Reps = 10
Weights = 8 pounds or more
Rest for 30 seconds in between sets

Tip: Extend both arms at the same time for an advanced workout.

Target Areas: Triceps (Arms)

Two Arm Row

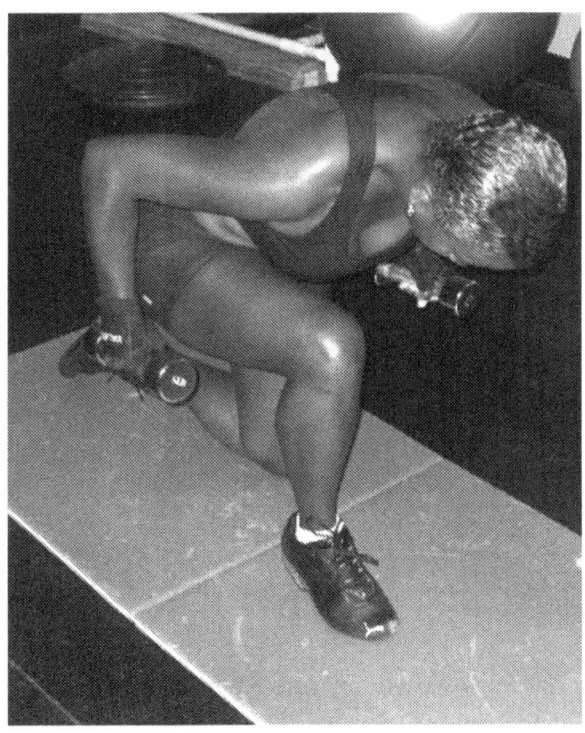

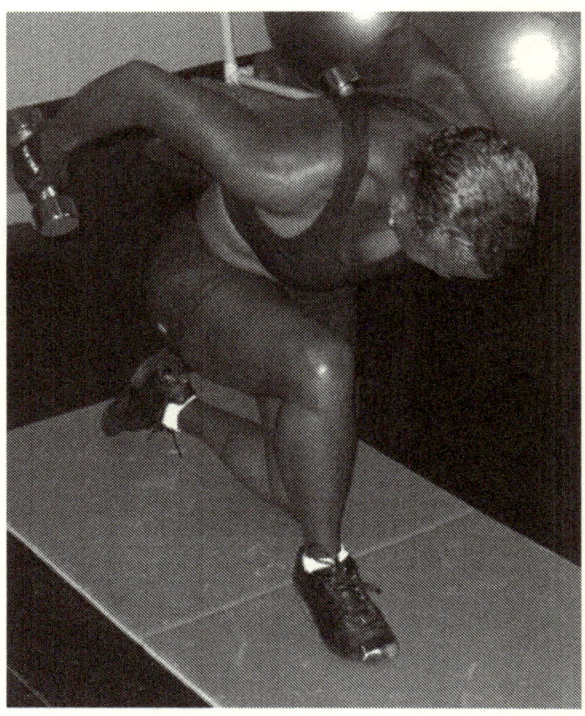

This exercise is great for conditioning the muscles in your upper back.

Steps:

1. Lower yourself down on one knee and lean your torso against your front leg.

2. Place the weights in your hands and extend your arms to the floor with your palms facing in.

3. Slowly pull your elbows back and inward as your hands separate.

4. Release your arms to their starting position.

5. Hold in your stomach to support your back.

6. Breathe.

Deconditioned routine
Sets = 1
Reps = 8 to 10
Weights = 3 to 5 pounds
Increase sets and reps after 3 weeks.

Tips: Sit in a chair instead of kneeling.
Keep your shoulder blades pulled down toward your waist.

Conditioned routine
Sets = 3
Reps = 10
Weights = 8 pounds or more
Rest for 30 seconds in between sets

Target Areas: (Trapezius) Upper back

Superman

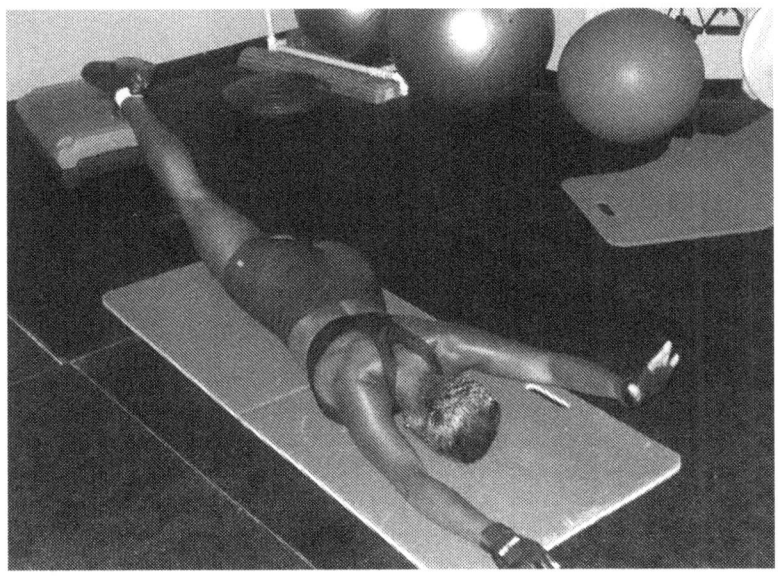

I love this one too, you get to work your butt and back at the same time!

Contraindications: Keep your head aligned with your spine. Do not arch your back. Control your movements and move slowly.

Steps:

1. Lie on the floor with your arms and legs extended.
2. Lift one arm and the opposite leg simultaneously away from the floor.
3. Release and repeat using the other arm and leg.
4. Hold your stomach in.
5. Breathe.

Deconditioned routine
Sets = 1
Reps = 8 to 10
Weights = 3 to 5 pounds (use to increase resistance)
Increase sets and reps after 3 weeks

Conditioned routine
Sets = 3
Reps = 10
Rest 30 seconds in between sets

Target Areas: Back and Gluteus

Side Raises

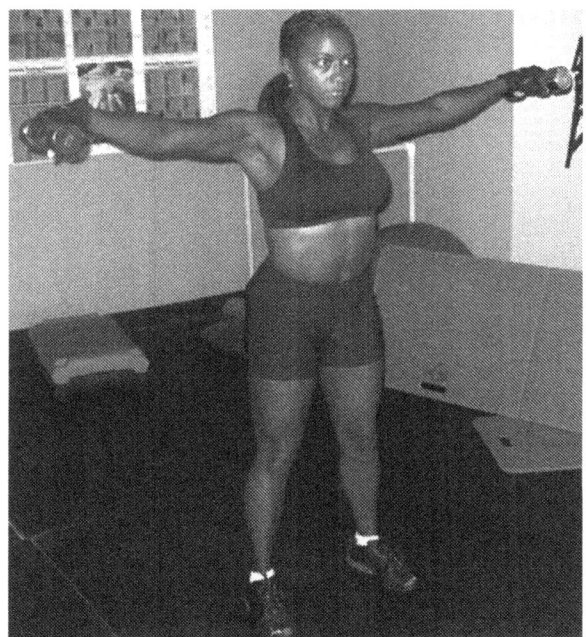

Contraindications: Do not swing the weights.
Do not lift the weights higher than shoulder level. Do not let the weights fall quickly. Keep your knees slightly bent.

Steps:

1. Stand with your feet hip-width apart and hold the dumbbells next to the sides of your legs, your palms should face in.

2. Slowly lift your arms out to your sides and away from your body and then release them. Do not lift the weights higher than your shoulder level.

3. Hold in your stomach to support your back.

4. Breathe

Deconditioned routine
Sets = 1
Reps = 8 to 10
Weights = 3 to 5 pounds
Increase sets and reps after 3 weeks.
Tip: Begin this exercise seated to help support your back.

Conditioned routine
Sets = 3
Reps = 10
Weights = 8 to 10 pounds
Rest for 30 seconds in between sets

Target Areas: Deltoids (Shoulders)

Overhead Press

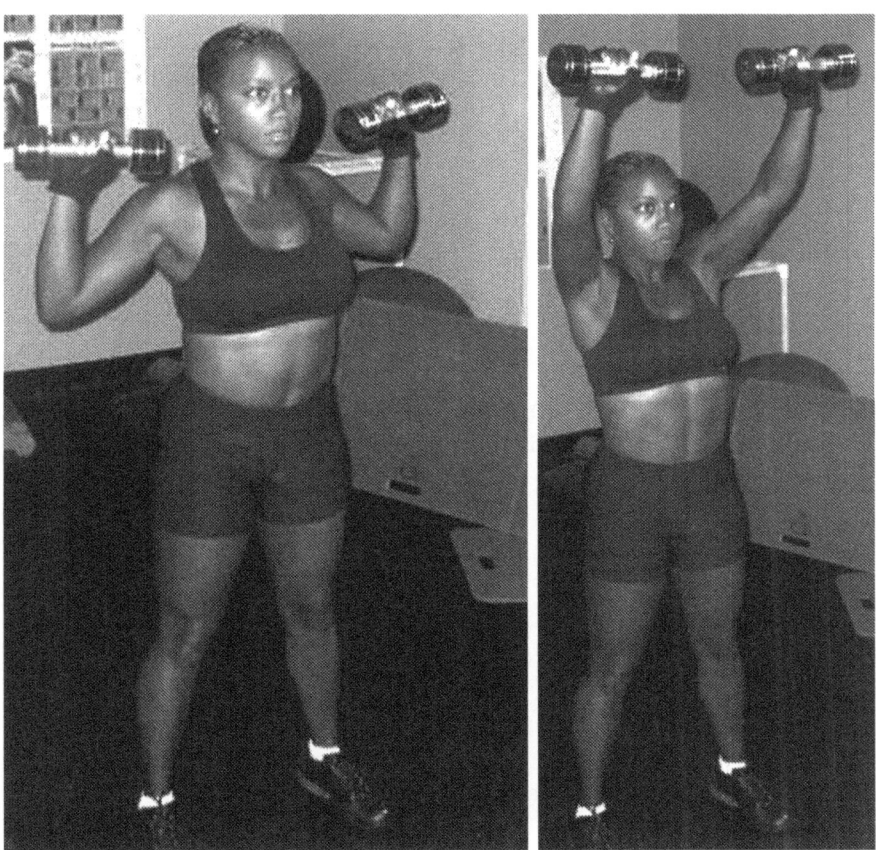

Begin with dumbbells in hands, just above the shoulders and aligned with your ears.

Contraindications: Keep your back straight. The weights should be in line with your ears not your face. If you experience shoulder pain, Stop, this may be an indication of an injury to your rotator cuff.

Steps:

1. Stand with your feet hip-width apart.

2.   Hold the dumbbells at your shoulders and next to your ears with your palms facing forward.

3.   Slowly extend the weight overhead as you straighten your arms, and then release your arms back down to your shoulder level.

4.   Hold in your stomach to support your back.

5.   Breathe!

Deconditioned routine
Sets = 1
Reps = 8 to 10
Weights = 3 to 5 pounds
Increase sets and reps after 3 weeks.
Tip: Sit on a chair with your feet staggered and flat on the floor to support your back.

Conditioned routine
Sets = 3
Reps = 10
Weights = 8 to 10 pounds
Rest for 30 seconds in between sets

Targeted Areas: Deltoids (Shoulders)

Let's move onto the lower body focusing first on the abdominal exercises. I love these they helped me get back into my clothes after two pregnancies! That was my goal, but everybody has their own personal reasons why they workout. Some desire a 6 pack, while others just want to keep their belly from rolling over the sides of their belts! Whatever your desire, it is tangible! You can achieve flatter more defined abdominal muscles too. Here are some facts about our abdominal muscles:
Did you know there are four types of abdominal muscles?
Rectus Abdominis—spans from the lowest point of the chest bone to the pelvic bone

Internal/External Obliques—run diagonally up and down the sides of the mid portion of your torso

Traverse Abdominis—this muscle contracts when you cough or sneeze.

Our abdominal muscles work as a team to help support the lower back and stabilize the torso. Our abdominals enable us to bend forward, backward, and rotate at the trunk of the body.

Word of advice, do not hold your breath while doing these exercises, the key is to exhale as you contract the muscles and inhale as you release. If you do it this way, you will be surprised at how many sit-ups you can do. There are several exercises for this group of muscles, but here are the ones I find most effective.

Curl Up

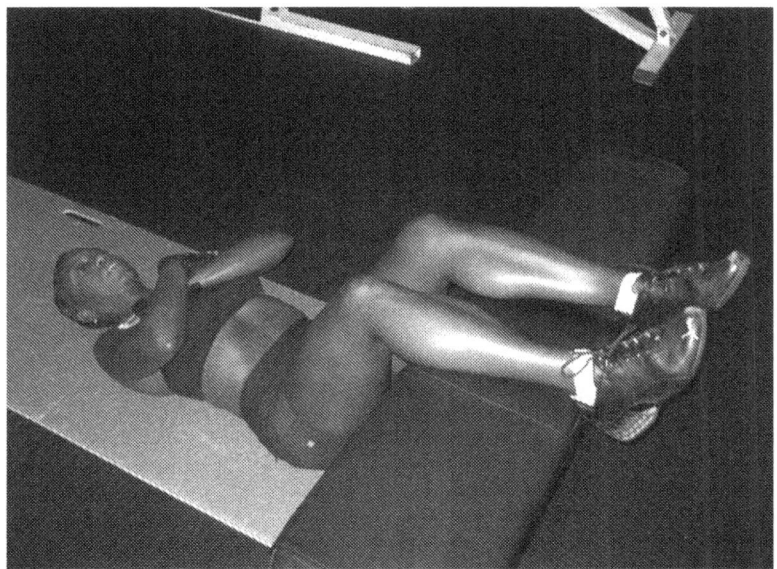

This exercise is very effective! I did this twice a day for 6 months, after giving birth. I gained a total of 135 pounds with both pregnancies, most of it in the stomach area. I worked like a dog to get my stomach down!

All you need to get started is a chair and the floor. The goal of this exercise is to see how high you can curl your torso, and to lift your shoulders off the floor high enough to feel your abdominals tighten.

Tip: Use a mat or a carpeted floor for comfort. Breathing is KEY! It is important to exhale during the period of contraction (on your way up from the floor).

Contraindications:
Do not place your hands behind your head; this will put emphasis on lifting your neck rather than working your abs. Keep your head and neck aligned with your spine. Keep your chin off your chest; pretend you have an orange between your chin and your chest. Maintain the strength of your abs throughout the movement to help prevent back injury.

Steps:

1. Lie on your back, rest your feet on a couch or chair, and place your arms across your chest.

2. Lift your head and shoulders off the floor as you lift your torso up toward the ceiling and in toward your hips.

3. Release your torso back to the floor in a slow controlled motion.

4. Exhale as you contract up and inhale as you resist down.

Deconditioned routine
Sets = 1
Reps = 10 or more
Increase your sets (max 3 after 3 weeks)

Conditioned routine
Sets = 3
Reps = 25
Rest for 30 seconds in between sets
Hold for three seconds as you lift up and one second to resist down

Target Areas: Hello, the Abs!

Side Slide

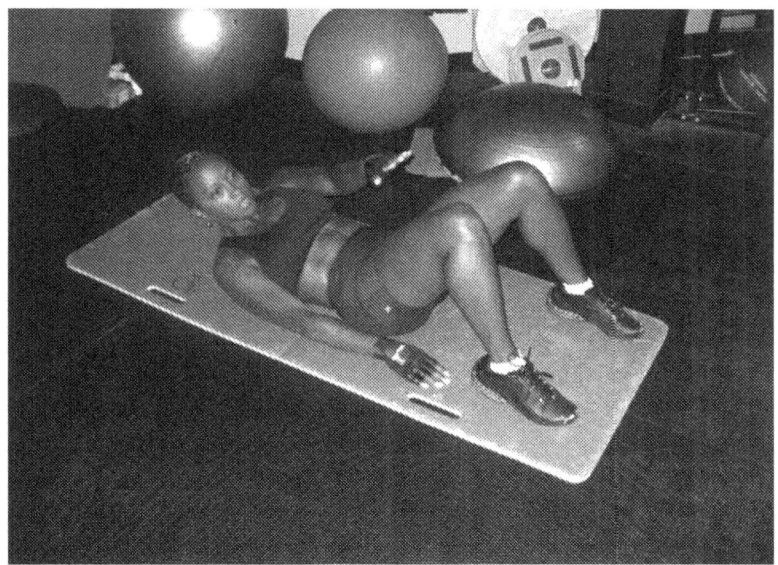

Simply slide from side to side. (Try saying that fast three times!)

Contraindications: Review the contraindications from the previous exercise.
Keep your lower back on the floor, no arching.

Steps:

1. Lie on your back with your knees bent and feet on the floor.

2. Place your right arm extended above in front of you and lift your shoulders slightly off the floor.

3. With your left hand, reach or slide down the side of your body toward your left heel contracting your oblique muscles.

4. Repeat your reaches, exhaling as you reach down and inhaling as you return to the center position.

5. Switch hands and repeat on the other side.

Deconditioned routine
Sets = 1
Reps = 10 on each side
Increase your sets (max 3 after 3 weeks)

Conditioned routine
Sets = 3
Reps = 20 on each side
Rest for 30 seconds in between sets
Hold for a count of three seconds as you lift up and one second to resist down

Target Areas: Obliques (Abs)

This next one is easy to do, ready, set, **laugh!**
Everyone should laugh at least once a day to relieve stress, so find something that cracks you up and have a great time working those abdominal muscles.

Moving right along let's discuss some ways to improve our legs!
Strong legs can take you a long way, think about it, we need them to get out of bed and carry our body weight around everyday. Whether you want to bike, run, swim, or walk, strong legs get you there faster. I'm not going to bore you with a million details about your legs, but here are a few basic facts about the muscle structure. Four major muscle groups make up the beauty that is our legs. They are the quadriceps, hamstrings, gastrocnemius and soleus, and tibialis anterior. The quads are the largest group of muscles in our body they provide power to the lower leg. The ham's purpose is to help pull your heel up to the back of your thigh. The hams come in handy when you need to run. Sprinters need loose hams to run at record—breaking speeds. In simpler terms, quads push and hams pull the muscles in

your legs. If you equally strengthen these pull and push muscles you will prevent injury to your knee joints and increase your stamina in cardio exercises. The gastrocnemius and soleus are located in the calf area. These muscles help you stand on the tips of your toes to feel taller and reach things. I'm 5 feet tall I use my calves to compare my height to my teenage sons, they have me beat by miles! We **laugh** (remember those abs!) about the height difference all of the time. The tibialis anterior or shin is located in the front of your lower leg. The shin's purpose is to lift the ball of your foot and plant your heel into the ground. When you walk, run or hike, you are exercising your shins, because your heels hit the ground before the balls of your feet.

The following are exercises for strong legs … ready here we go.

Squats

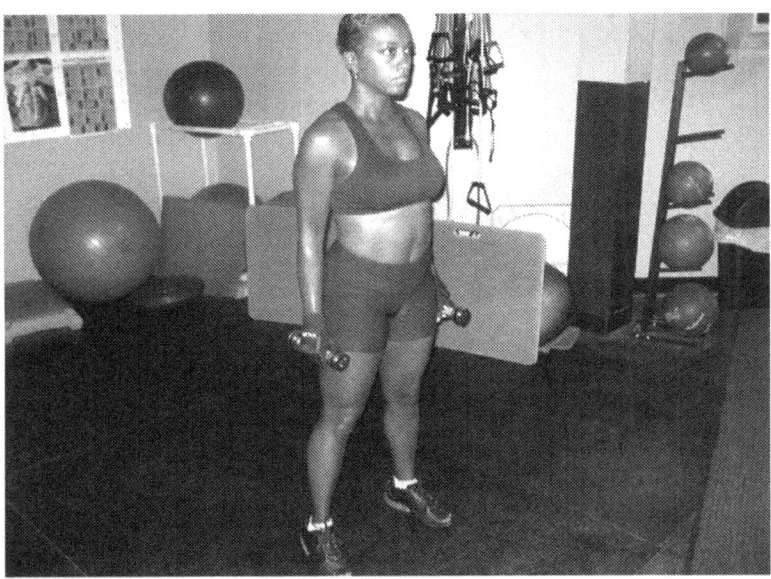

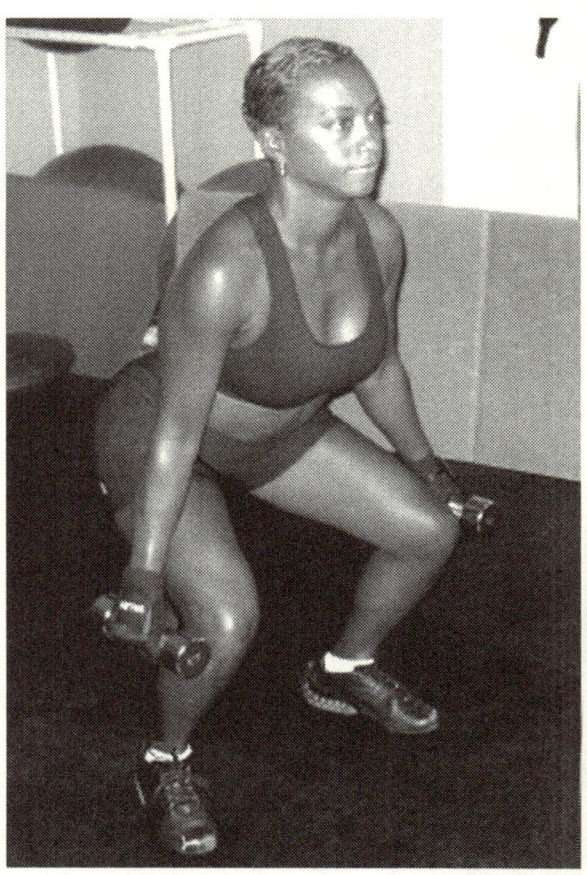

Use a mirror to check your form for the squat.
Note you will not go all the way down to the floor.

Contraindications: Make sure your knees do not extend past your toes as you lower yourself down. Tighten your abdominals to support your torso. Keep the weight of your body in your heels to work your buttocks and legs.

Steps:

1.   Stand with your feet hip-width apart. You may want to hold onto something for balance and support such as a chair.

2. Slowly lower your body downward by pushing your buns backward. I want you to sit in a chair.

3. Push your weight back up by pressing from your heels and extend your body up to your starting position.

4. Breathe!

Deconditioned routine
Sets = 1
Reps = 8 to 10
Weights = 0 to 3 lbs
Increase your sets (max 3 after 3 weeks)

Tip: For help place a chair under your buns and lower yourself as far as you can.

Conditioned routine
Sets = 3
Reps = 10
Weights = 5 to 10 lbs.
Rest for 30 seconds in between sets
Hold five seconds as you lift up.

Target Areas: Quads, hams and buttocks

Double Leg Extensions

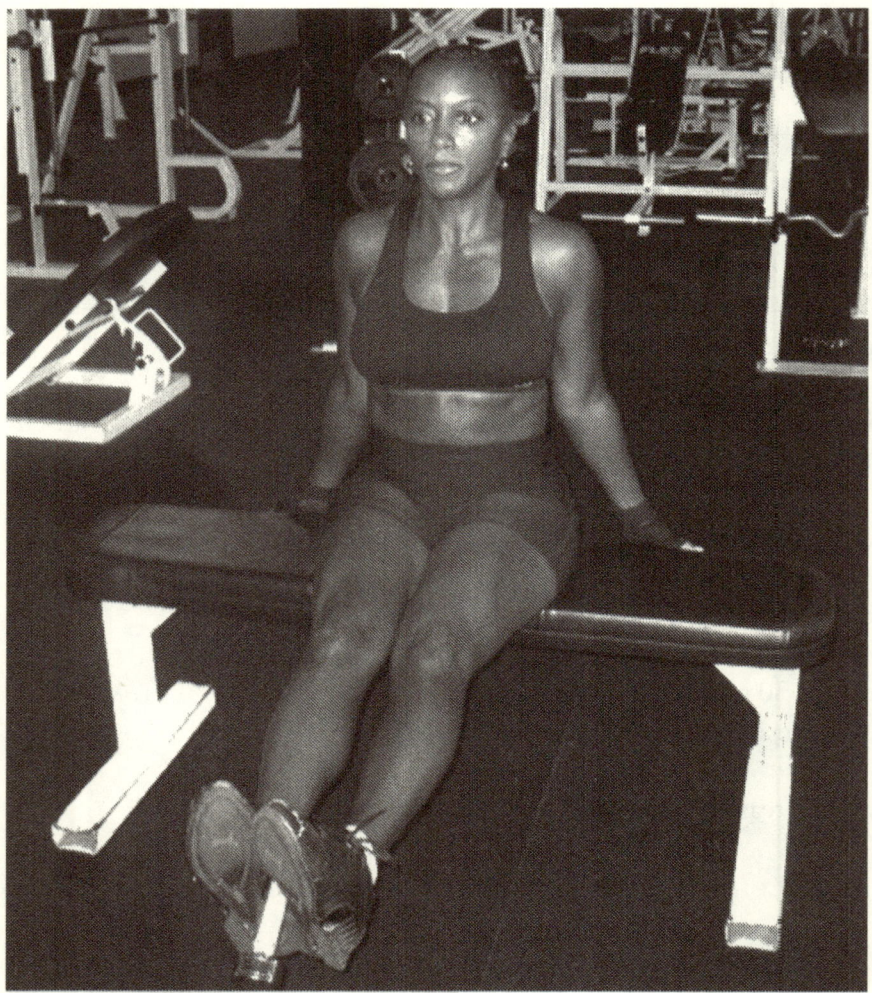

This exercise is very effective but it is not a pleasurable experience. I prefer the squat, but it is always great to have an alternative. If you are just beginning to work out I do not recommended that you try this exercise with weights. Once your legs feel strong, slowly add weight.

Contraindications: Work slowly and with control throughout the exercise. Maintain a straight torso with your abs pulled in to support your back. Do not continue this exercise if you experience knee pain.

Steps:

1. Sit near the edge of a chair or a couch with your hands holding the seat and your feet barely touching the floor.

2. Place the dumbbell (if you are using weights) between your feet, squeezing your feet together to hold it in place.

3. Slowly extend both knees, taking your feet straight out and up.

4. Squeeze your quads at the top of the motion and then release your legs to their starting position.

5. Breathe!

Deconditioned routine
Sets = 1
Reps = 8 to 10
Weights = 0 to 3 lbs
Increase your sets (max 3 after 3 weeks)

Conditioned routine
Sets = 3
Reps = 10
Weights = 5 to 8 lbs
Rest for 30 seconds in between sets
Change your count to lift feet up in 3 seconds and resist down in 1 second

Target Areas: Quads and Abs

Single Leg Heel Curl

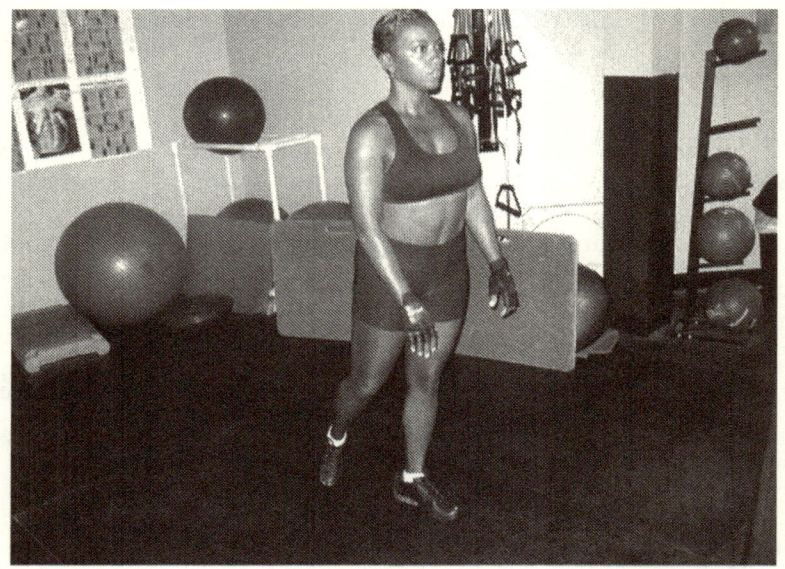

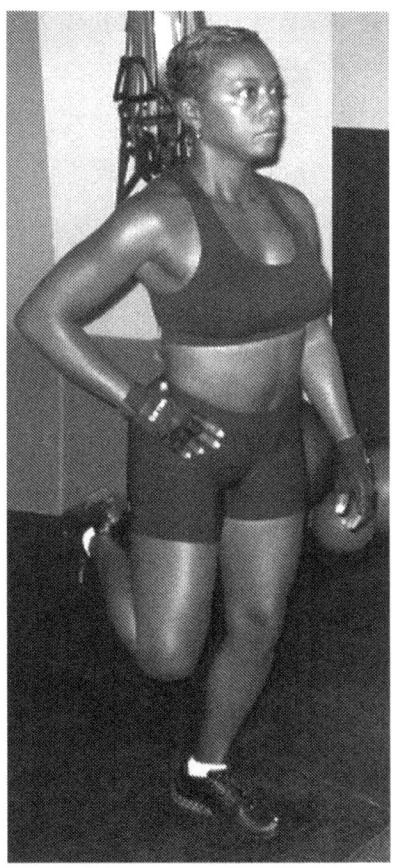

This exercise will strengthen the hamstrings.

Contraindications:

Be sure to keep the knee of your supporting leg (the one you are balancing on) slightly bent. Do not LOCK your knee joint. Squeeze your hams and buns as you contract your leg so that you do not lean forward. Maintain alignment of your head, shoulders, and hips with your supporting leg.

Steps:

1. Stand on one leg with the other leg extended behind you.

2. Bend your knee so that your foot comes up behind you and slowly lift your heel up to your buns.

3. Bring your foot back down to the floor slowly and repeat.

4. Switch legs and continue the exercise with the other leg.

5. Breathe!

Deconditioned routine

Sets = 1
Reps = 8 to 10 each leg
Increase your sets (max 3 after 3 weeks)

Tip: Hold a chair for support.

Conditioned routine
Sets = 3
Reps = 10 to 12 each leg
Rest for 30 seconds in between sets
To add resistance, use ankle weights and change your count to lift up in 3 seconds and resist down in 1 second

Target Areas: Hamstrings

First Position: (heels together, toes out)

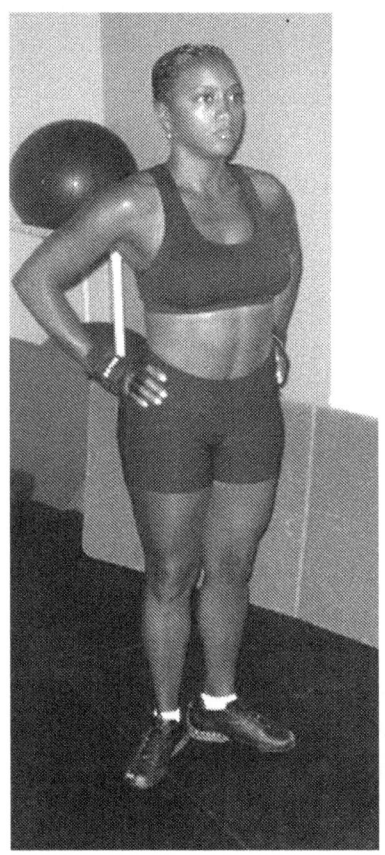 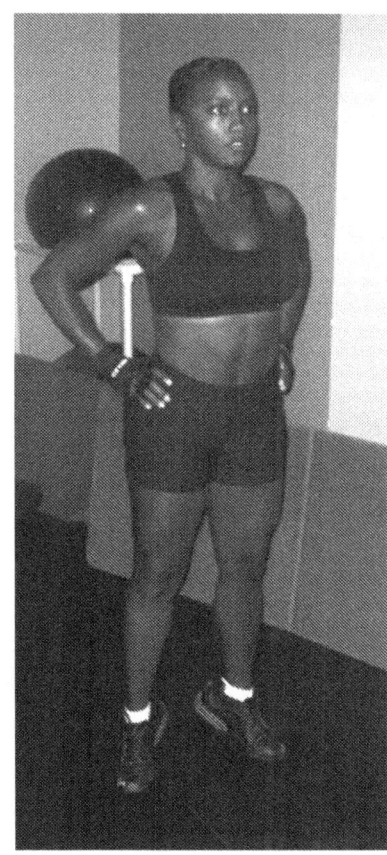

For stronger calves, try this exercise.

Contraindications: Keep your knees straight and work strictly through your ankles and feet. Control your movement being careful not to rock back and forth.

Steps:

1. Stand with your heels touching and toes angles outward at a 45-degree angle.

2.   Slowly raise your body onto the balls of your feet.

3.   Squeeze your calves at the top of your lift and then release back down to the floor.

4.   Breathe!

Deconditioned routine
Sets = 1
Reps = 10 to 12 each leg
Increase your sets (max 3 after 3 weeks)

Tip: Hold a chair for support.

Conditioned routine
Sets = 3
Reps = 15 to 20 each leg

To add resistance, add a dumbbell to the workout
Rest for 30 seconds in between sets

Target Areas: Calves

Ankle Rolls

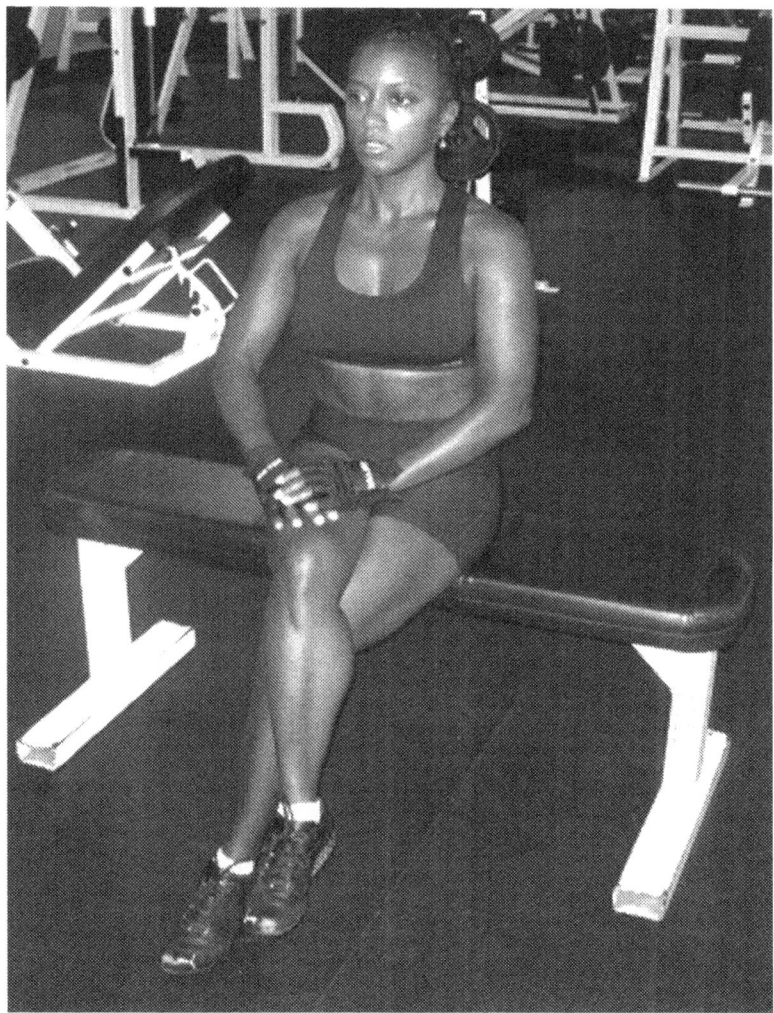

You can do this while waiting or sitting at your desk.

Contraindications: Sit up straight to support your back. Control your movement to avoid rocking back and forth.

Steps:

1. Sit in a chair with one leg crossed over the other.

2. Fold your hands over your knees. This will hinder your leg from moving.

3. Slowly rotate your foot in circles (in both directions) by contracting your lower leg muscles. Make full circles with your foot.

Deconditioned routine
Sets = 1
Reps = 10 each leg
Increase your sets (max 3 after 3 weeks)

Conditioned routine
Sets = 2
Reps = 10 each leg

Target Areas: Shins

The next set of exercises will help you firm your thighs! Most of us hate the fat that surrounds the thigh muscles. If your thighs jiggle it does not mean your muscles are weak, it means fat is covering the muscles. The two major muscles we are concerned about are the adductors located in the inner side of your hips and thighs, because they align your legs with the midline of your body, and the abductors located along the outer side of your hips and thighs, these muscles pull your legs away from the center of your body. We need both sets of muscles for balance while riding a bike, horse, skiing or skating. For those of you who play tennis, volleyball, golf, baseball, and boxing, you have noticed that strong thighs give you the ability to change directions and transfer your weight.

The following exercises will work your thighs (I love these!)

Inner Thigh Side Lifts

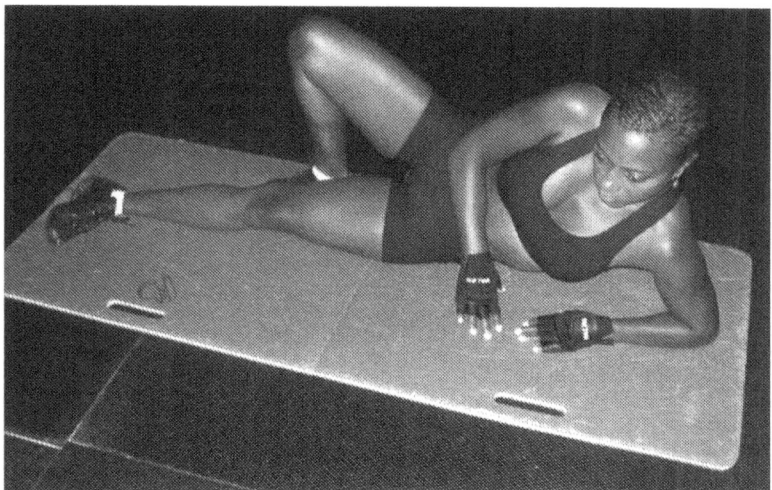

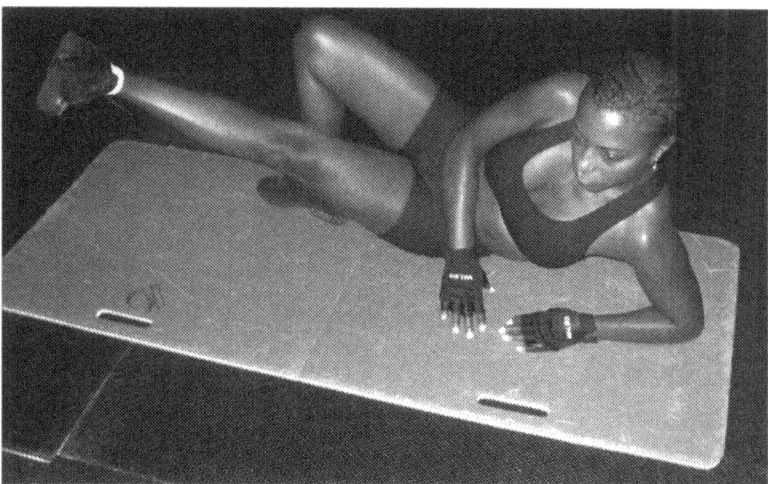

For an effective workout concentrate on squeezing your adductor muscles while lifting your leg. If you want to increase the intensity, put an ankle weight on the leg you are lifting.

Contraindications: Do not swing your leg up and down. Your movements should be slow and controlled. Lift your heel up toward the ceiling to focus on adductor muscles. Keep your abdominals tight as you lift your leg.

Steps:

1. Lie on a carpet or covered floor for added cushion.

2. Lie on your side and first place your top leg behind the bottom leg.

3. Prop yourself up on one elbow or extend your arm and rest your head on that arm.

4. Lift the foot of your bottom leg (which is straight) and raise it toward the ceiling, then slowly lower it to the floor.

5. Repeat with the other leg.

6. Breathe!

Note: Fully extend the bottom leg

Deconditioned routine
Sets = 1
Reps = 8 to 10 each leg
Increase your sets (max 3 after 3 weeks)

Conditioned routine
Sets = 3
Reps = 15 to 20 each leg

Target Areas: Inner Thigh (Adductors) and Abs!

Standing Side Leg Lift

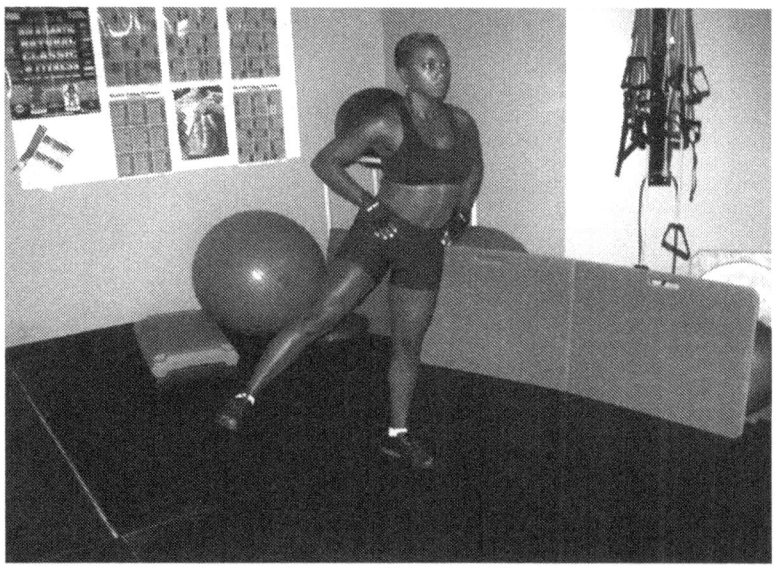

If standing is your thing, this exercise is for you. This exercise will work your abductors (outer thighs).

Contraindications: Keep the knee of your base leg slightly bent, do not lock your knee joint. Keep your knees facing forward and your abdominals tight. Lift your legs with slow and controlled movements.

Steps:

1. Stand on one leg (base leg) with the other leg just touching the floor with the ball of your foot. Note: the leg barely touching the floor is your working leg.

2. Keeping your body straight, slowly raise the working leg outward.

3. Release and repeat using your other leg as the working leg.

4. Breathe!

Deconditioned routine
Sets = 1
Reps = 10 each leg
Increase your sets (max 3 after 3 weeks)

Tip: Hold onto a chair for balance.

Conditioned routine
Sets = 3
Reps = 10 to 15 each leg
Add an ankle weight to your working leg for more resistance and increased difficulty.

Target Areas: Abductors (outer thighs) and abs

Now lets' discuss the largest single muscle in our body the gluteus maximus!
Also known as the buns, cheeks and in some circles the bubble butt. Having a bubble butt is not necessarily a bad thing. The important thing is firmness not size. We do not want any jiggle (cellulite) in the butt area. The exercises below will definitely work your butt into shape!

Tip: The key to maximizing your results is to keep your weight in your heels during the leg and bun exercises.

Butt Burning Lunges

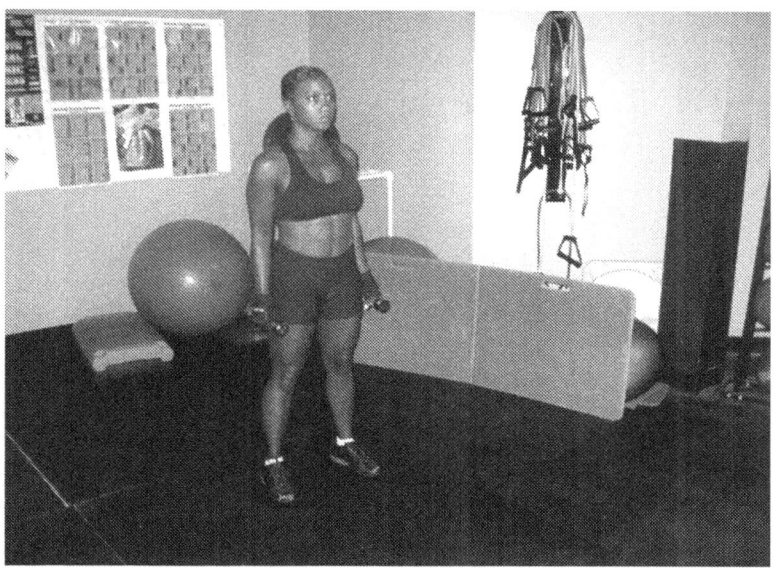

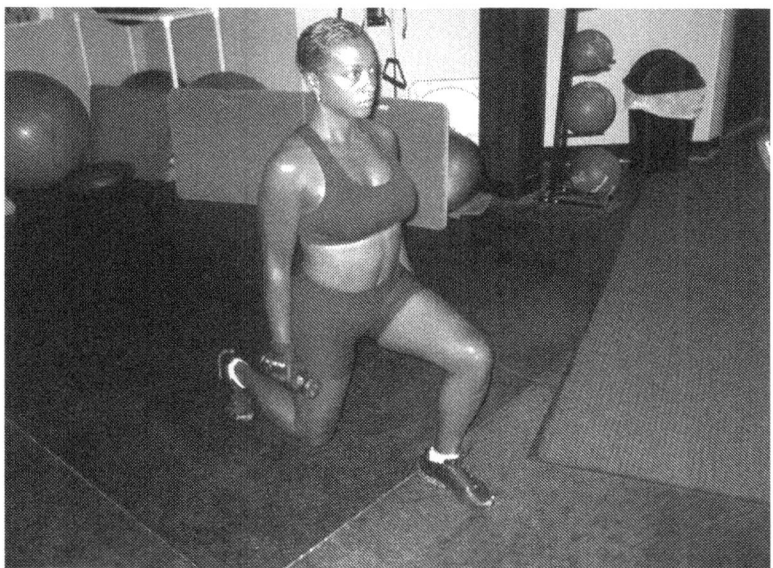

This exercise is easy and yields results!

Contraindications: Do not allow your knee to extend past your toes. Flex your knee at a 90-degree angle. Keep your weight in your front heel to focus on the butt. Do not bend at the waist keep your torso straight throughout the movement. Tighten your abs to support your back.

Steps:

1. Stand with your feet together and hands resting on your hips.

2. Carefully step forward with one leg and lower your body down to the floor. Your knee should never touch the floor.

3. Keep your front knee aligned over your front ankle and maintain your weight in your front heel.

4. Push yourself back to your starting position with your front foot.

5. Alternate legs.

6. Breathe!

Deconditioned routine
Sets = 1
Reps = 8 each leg
Increase your sets (max 3 after 3 weeks)

Conditioned routine
Sets = 3
Reps = 10 each leg
Tip: Hold dumbbells for added intensity.

Target Areas: Buttocks

Rear Leg Lifts

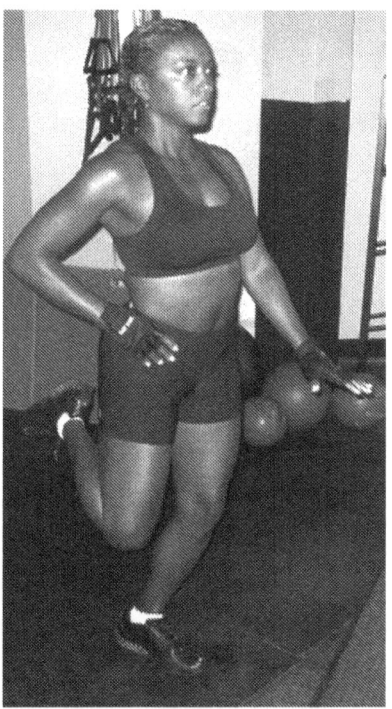

This exercise will lift your buns for sure. For more resistance, add an ankle weight to the leg you are lifting.

Contraindications: Do not swing your leg. Squeeze your butt and tighten your abs as you lift your leg. Keep your base knee slightly bent; be careful not lock your knee joint.

Steps:

1. Stand up straight with your feet placed shoulder width apart. Place one foot (working leg) behind you. Your other leg remains as your support leg (base leg).

2. Keeping both of your knees slightly bent, lift your working leg toward the ceiling without arching your back.

3. Squeeze your butt as you lift and slowly release your leg back to the floor.

4. Repeat with the other leg.

5. Breathe!

Deconditioned routine
Sets = 1
Reps = 10 each leg
Increase your sets (max 3 after 3 weeks)

Tip: Hold onto a chair for balance.

Conditioned routine
Sets = 3
Reps = 10 each leg
Add an ankle weight to your working leg for resistance and increased difficulty.

Target Areas: Buttocks and abs

Rear End Tilts

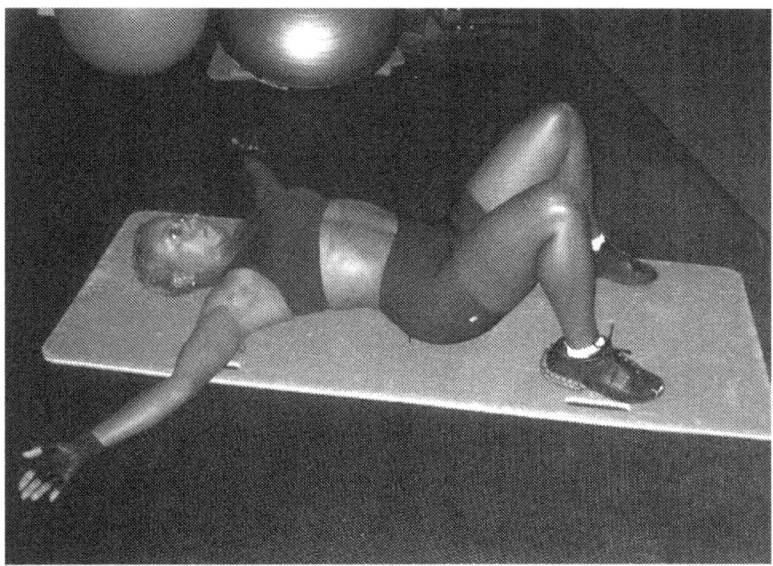

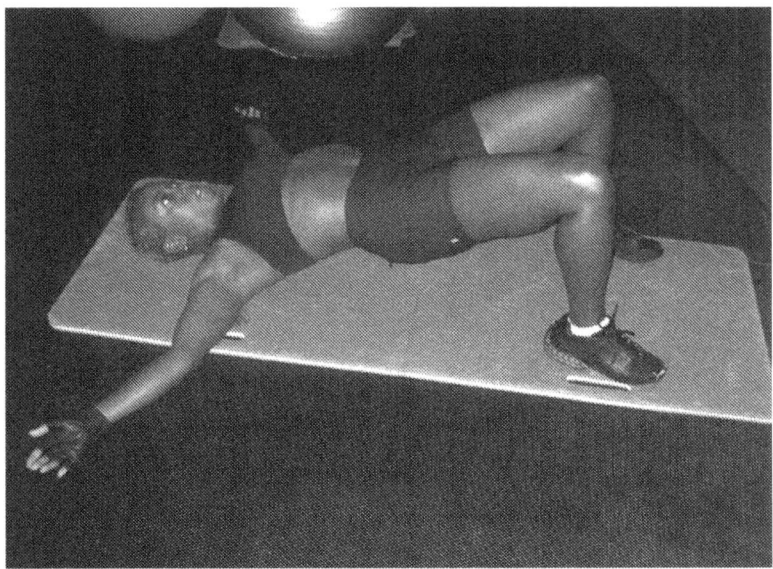

You can do this while watching the news or your favorite TV program.

Contraindications: Tighten your abdominals as you elevate your hips in order to support your back.

Steps:

1. Lie on your back with your knees bent, your feet flat on the floor, and your arms extended at each side.

2. Press your weight up from your heels to elevate your hips off the floor.

3. Concentrate on squeezing your butt as you move through the motion.

4. Slowly lower yourself to the floor and repeat.

5. Breathe!

Deconditioned routine
Sets = 1
Reps = 10
Increase your sets (max 3 after 3 weeks)

Conditioned routine
Sets = 3
Reps = 10 to 12
Target Areas: Buttocks and abs

Whew! What a work out! Since, we can't achieve the health we are striving for eating like the cookie monster and the hamburglar. Let's move on to discuss ways to nourish our bodies without washing all of our workout efforts down the drain.

"Keep winking, I'm already thinking I've got it going on!"

Chapter 4: Uummm Good and Good For Me!

I have to start this chapter with an introduction dedicated to our body's best friend WATER. Water is essential to the human body's survival. We can live for about a month without food, but only about a week without water. Water and its benefits are highly beneficial to the human body. Water can help us maintain a healthy body weight by increasing metabolism and regulating appetite, which in turn leads to increased energy levels. Did you know that most day-time fatigue is actually mild dehydration? Water naturally moisturizes the skin and ensures proper cellular formation underneath the layers of skin providing a healthy, glowing appearance. With that in mind, it is safe to say that water supports beauty from the inside out! Drinking water regularly not only helps to decrease the risk of cancers such as; breast, colon and bladder, by flushing out disease causing waste and bacteria. It also helps to reduce headaches and urinary tract infections, relieve joint and back pain and prevent constipation. To sum it up, water is crucial to our fitness, because a properly hydrated body functions at its peak!

*Fact: Water is the only drink that will thoroughly flush toxins from the body and help you lose weight.

Calculating your proper water intake is simple using the following equation.

Your weight divided by two = your proper water intake

For example if you weigh 150 pounds, your daily water intake is 150 divided by 2, which equals 75oz. Like most people, you probably don't count ounces or the number of glasses of water you drink a day. An easy solution is to purchase a water bottle with the measurements on the side. As a result, you will begin to monitor your intake, because you will have to refill it throughout the day. Another suggestion is to drink your daily consumption through a straw. Instead of gulping directly from a cup, the straw will make it easier to consume larger amounts of water, it also it looks better for those in a professional setting.

*Facts: If you eat a meal high in fat and salt, it is best to drink warm water with your meal, this helps your body to break the food down more effectively.

*Tip: Never exceed 128 oz in one day. Drinking too much water can cause an electrolyte imbalance and ultimately water poisoning leading to fatality.

After a workout, you're going to be hungry and I'm sure you don't want to nibble on a carrot you want to EAT! Thankfully, developing healthy eating habits does not mean you have to starve. In order to reap the benefits of our hard work, it is important to understand how to eat delicious meals without packing on the pounds. Lets start with the food pyramid. The food pyramid is one of the easiest ways to understand how to eat healthy. The USDA updated it in the spring of 2005 to assist Americans with making healthier choices. The chart consists of rainbow colored vertical stripes, which represent the five food groups plus fats and oils.

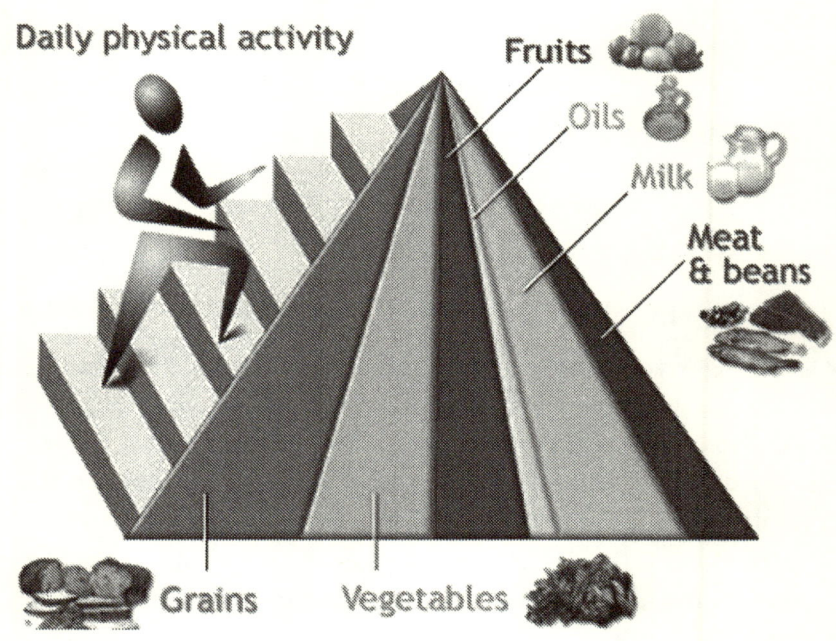

Here's what the colors stand for:

- orange—grains
- green—vegetables
- red—fruits
- yellow—fats and oils
- blue—milk and dairy products
- purple—meat, beans, fish, and nuts

How colorful is your plate?

Notice the steps on the side of the pyramid they symbolize the small steps we have to take to healthy nourishment. Let's discuss some of the other messages this chart is trying to communicate.

Eat a variety of foods. A balanced diet is one that includes all the food groups. In other words, have foods from every color, every day.

Eat less of some and more of others. The bands for meat, protein (purple) and oils (yellow) are smaller than the others, because our bodies need less of those foods. The bands are wider at the base and thinner as they approach the top. This chart cleverly tells us that all-foods-are-not-created equal, even within a healthy food group like fruit. For example, apple pie would be in that thin part of the fruit band because it has a lot of added sugar and fat. On the other hand, an apple (crunch!) would be in the wider area, because they contain natural sugars allowing us to eat them without feeling guilty.

Grains

Ounce equivalents are used to measure grain. Here are some ounce equivalents for common grain foods. An ounce equivalent equals:

- 1 piece of bread
- 1/2 cup of cooked cereal, like oatmeal

- 1/2 cup of rice or pasta
- 1 cup of cold cereal

And one last thing about grains: Try to eat a lot of whole grains, such as 100% wheat bread, brown rice, and oatmeal. Consume up to 6 oz daily.

Vegetables

We need vegetables especially those dark green and orange ones. Vegetable servings are measured in cups. It's best to consume between 1-2 cups of veggies per day.

Fruits

Sweet, juicy fruit is definitely part of a healthy diet. Consume between 1-1 ½ cups of fruit daily.

Milk and Other Calcium-Rich Foods

Calcium builds strong bones, so we need these foods in our diet. If you aren't a big fan of milk, you can substitute with yogurt, cheese, or calcium fortified orange juice—just to name a few. Consume between 1-3 servings per day.

Meats, Beans, Fish, and Nuts

These foods contain iron and other healthy body nutrients. These foods like grains are measured in ounce equivalents as well. Examples of ounce equivalents for this group are:

- 1 ounce of meat, poultry, or fish
- 1/4 cup cooked dry beans
- 1 egg
- 1 tablespoon of peanut butter
- a small handful of nuts or seeds

Just remember those stairs climbing up the side of the new pyramid, taking it one-step at a time. Now that we know which foods to eat and how much, lets discuss how to read labels, so we can make educated choices in the grocery store.

Nonfat Milk
Serving Size 8 fl oz (240mL)
Servings Per Container 2

Amount Per Serving

Calories 80	Calories from Fat 0

% Daily Value*

Total Fat 0g	0%
Saturated Fat 0g	0%
Cholesterol less than 5mg	1%
Sodium 130mg	5%
Total Carbohydrate 12g	4%
Dietary Fiber 0g	0%
Sugars 11g	

Protein 8g

Vitamin A 8%	•	Vitamin C 4%

Calcium 30% • Iron 0% • Vitamin D 25%

* Percent Daily Values are based on a 2,000 calorie diet. Your daily values may be higher or lower depending on your calorie needs.

		Calories:	2,000	2,500
Total Fat	Less than		65g	80g
Sat Fat	Less than		20g	25g
Cholesterol	Less than		300mg	300mg
Sodium	Less than		2,400mg	2,400mg
Total Carbohydrate			300g	375g
Dietary Fiber			25g	30g

Source: Food Packaging

1. **Watch Your Serving Size:** This example says two servings per package, so the information provided stands for only half the package.

2. **Check calories:** Put calories in perspective. Most meals are 300 to 400 calories and snacks 100 to 200.

3. **Watch the risky fats:** Limit your daily saturated and trans fats, to 15g for saturated and 1.6 g for trans fats. You can also choose to eliminate them. In addition, limit cholesterol to 300 mg and sodium to 2,300 mg

4. **Watch Your Carbs:** Women should aim for 25 g or more dietary fiber daily. Fiber is a natural occurring sugar in fruit and dairy products so it is safe, but like all sweets should be limited. If you are trying to lose weight, dietary fiber is your friend! Try to consume 25g of this slimming disease fighter daily.

5. **Protein:** Daily protein should be 60 g on a 1,200-calorie plan, 75 g and 90 g on 1,500 and 1,800-calorie plans, respectively.

6. **% Daily Value:** Keep in mind that these are rough guidelines based on the government recommended 2,000-calorie intake a day. This is too many calories to consume if your goal is to lose weight. The diet I provided is only 1200 calories.

7. **% Daily Value of vitamins and minerals:** This section provides a good way to compare relative levels of important nutrients, like calcium, among different products. Note: overly high levels of some vitamins and minerals are not always desirable.

Be aware of Fat, Salt and Carbs

The National Academy of Sciences says fat consumption should be 20 to 35 percent of your daily calories. However, the most important thing is to be aware of the amount of saturated and trans-fat in food. Diets heavy in saturated fat raise the blood pressure and cholesterol, increasing the risk of heart disease and stroke. Animal-based foods, such as butter, chicken skin and oils such as palm and coconut contain saturated fat naturally. Are you thinking, "Wow, I want nothing to do with that stuff"? Well, check this out; we cannot escape saturated fat even "good" oils like olive and canola contain small amounts of it. A heart healthy diet should have less than 10 percent of the total calories from saturated fat, which is a maximum of 12 g and 15 g saturated fat daily on 1,200 and 1,500-calorie diets. There's more bad news, trans fat (appearing as partially hydrogenated vegetable oil on labels) is worse than saturated fat, it raises LDL (bad cholesterol) and lowers HDL (good cholesterol) increasing heart complications. Try to keep your trans fat intake as low as possible.

Cholesterol is a fat like substance naturally made by our bodies and taken in through consumption, usually in foods of animal origin. The recommended daily limit is 300mg for the general population and 200mg for those with high cholesterol.

Sodium is not our friend! Yes, it adds flavor to food, but it also causes our body to retain water and happily contributes to heart disease by raising the blood pressure. The latest government recommendation is to have no more than 2,300 mg daily this amounts to a little less than a teaspoon per day. I know that sounds impossible, but look at the labels on soup and frozen dinners, some of these foods contain up to 1,000 mg of sodium!

Despite what most diets say, carbs are not our enemy. The key is to choose good carbs like whole wheat and rye breads, crackers, cereals, fruits, veggies, and oats (My entire family consumes oatmeal for breakfast, it provides the necessary carbs and helps to reduce cholesterol). Some frozen foods contain good carbs too. Here's how you can tell. The ingredients list will start with "good" carbs. It is always wise to avoid brands that start with sweeteners and white flour. Total carbs have three components: starch, sugar, and dietary fiber. There is no daily value for sugar, but the less sugar the better. We also need to limit added sugar from sweeteners. Ideally, we should have no more than 24g of added sugar per day this is equivalent to 6 teaspoons! One can of soda has 33g of sugar, so, put your hands up and walk away from the soda! What do you know about protein? Protein is the key to the growth of hormones, enzymes, and tissues. Our bodies break down the protein we consume, turning it into amino acids, the building blocks of all proteins. To get an adequate intake of protein we can consume a number of things such as: meat, chicken, fish, tofu, eggs, cheese, yogurt, and milk. While incomplete proteins such as leafy greens, grains, and most legumes, only contain some. As with all foods too much protein is unhealthy, so be aware of your daily intake.

Beware of Label Gimmicks

This is where many of us are misinformed. The only advice I have is to beware of the common phrases found on many food packages.

- **Cholesterol Free or No Cholesterol**—Take a look at canola oil its label says "NO CHOLESTEROL". Is this to say that the next brand without this claim is not as good? Remember our facts about cholesterol only foods of animal origin harbor cholesterol. This is a clever marketing ploy canola oil will never contain cholesterol.

- **Light**—This word can be used to describe fat content, taste, or color, and it is not always crystal clear as to which is being described. If the manufacturer is describing the fat content as "light", the product has at least 50% less fat than the original. The manufacturer must also state the fat percentage on the label, as in "50% less fat than our regular product". So don't get tricked into thinking that the word "light" necessarily means that you are getting a healthier product! Unless the label says that calories, fat, or sodium have been reduced, from the original product, you are not getting a health benefit.

- **Low fat or Fat free**—By law, these products have to be lower in fat than the original or virtually fat free. The key is to check the calories plenty of people have gained weight from eating too many fat free cookies and cakes, foods that are full of starch and sugar.

- **Low Sodium or Light in Sodium—Means** the sodium was reduced by at least half the original product. Super high sodium food such as soy sauce or even some soups although, listed as low sodium, still have large amounts of sodium. You can eat these foods, but make sure to factor their sodium level into your daily routine.

- **Sugar-free, No added sugars, With-out added sugars**—Ok, you will not believe this but the sugar-free chocolate on the shelf may not have a speck of sugar, but it still has plenty of fat and calories. Remember to always turn the package around and find out how may calories and grams of saturated fat you are consuming.

- **Sweetened with fruit juice, Fruit Juice Sweetener, or Fruit Juice Concentrate**-Boiling juice makes sweeteners—usually grape juice into a sticky sweetener. They may contain small amounts of potassium, don't get it twisted, they are not at all nutritious. These sweeteners are just like sugar!

Understanding the "Whole Grain" Craze!

According to the research at Harvard University, whole grain eaters are thinner than people who eat few whole grain foods and more processed white flour. Check this out, the Harvard study tracked 74,091 women for the past 10 years and found that women eating mostly whole grains weighed less than those who consumed the fewest. Those eating the whole grain ate 1.62 servings per 1,000 calories that is the equivalent to three servings of whole grains per day. The lowest consumers ate virtually no whole grains. Over the ten—year span, women who ate the mostly whole grains and other sources of dietary fiber gained less weight than those who ate the least. Researchers speculate that the whole grains may beneficially influence hormonal controls of weight, such as reducing insulin, which may decrease fat storage. In other studies, eating more whole grains is linked to a reduced risk of heart disease, diabetes, and certain types of cancer. The latest government recommendations: at least half of your grains should be whole-grain, which means at a minimum of 90 percent whole grains. Do you want to lose weight? Consume whole grain foods, I will tell you how to spot *real* whole grain! Here we go:

- Look for "whole" in the ingredient list. If you see, "whole-wheat", or "whole-rye", then it is clear the food contains whole grain.

- If it is called: brown rice, buckwheat, bulgur, cracked wheat, millet, quinoa, sorghum, wheat berries, whole grain barley, whole-grain corn, whole oats or oatmeal, wild rice, whole rye, whole wheat it is a whole grain.

- Corn flour, cornmeal, enriched flour, multigrain, (this means it is composed of various grains, not necessarily whole), pumpernickel, rice, rice flour, rye flour or rye, stoned ground wheat, wheat (alone), wheat flour, wheat germ, (not a whole grain, but it is still good for you, my husband eats this one!) and unbleached wheat flour none of these are whole grains.

- Look to see where the whole grain falls in the ingredient list. Foods are listed in order of weight, starting with the heaviest, so if a whole grain is the only ingredient listed, there is a lot of whole grain! We usually find wheat-flour (white flour) listed as the first ingredient, followed by a sweetener. In this case whole grain is not the dominant grain, there may only be a trace amount.

- Check dietary fiber. In general, 100 percent whole grain bread should have at least 2 grams fiber per ounce per 80 calories; crackers at least 3 grams fiber per ounce; pasta at least 5 grams per 2 ounces dried.

- Beware of labels that claim, "Made with Whole Grain". This means a little whole grain is included, but white flour is primarily the main ingredient.

Americans tend to have eating habits that are high in fat and protein. Food is now processed and more contaminated than ever before, causing us to suffer alarmingly from degenerative diseases such as heart disease, stroke, high blood pressure and diabetes. As a result, physicians have brought attention to the link between good health and nutrition. I urge you to stay away from stressor foods, they make us feel satisfied, but they do not provide nourishment for the body.

Stressor Foods (Foods with High Fat Content)
Cheeseburger—45%
Potato Chips—60%
Cheddar Cheese—74%
Beef Steak, untrimmed—74%
Whole Milk—40%
Chicken—24%
Beef Frank—82%
Mayonnaise—99%

Instead, move towards an optimal diet "whole foods" consisting of a variety of colored vegetables, fruits, whole grains, butter, and beans.

Do you need more energy?

It seems like we are always looking for a faster and easier way to lose weight, tone up, and be healthy. Remember this is a life style change so you need to be patient with yourself. I urge you to beware of gimmicks and plans that tell you to take pills, mix powders, or digest concoctions to obtain more energy. The truth is there are basic high-energy foods that give us the power we need to fuel our workouts and lives.
As we discussed earlier a good diet includes the four basic nutrients: Carbs, proteins, fats, and water.

Dark Green Leafy Vegetables—spinach, kale, and baby greens are good sources of free radical fighting anti-oxidants and calcium, which plays an important role in keeping muscles toned during exercise. It also helps maintain peak bone mass. Cruciferous veggies like broccoli, cabbage, and brussel sprouts (which by the way are not my favorite), are loaded with antioxidants that pack a punch against aging and may help to prevent cancer.

Whole grains—whole-wheat breads and crackers are great sources of fiber and B vitamins. Fiber-rich grains release energy to working muscles, giving you a sustained workout fuel when combined with protein and fat. These tan colored carbs also help balance hormones.

Beans—I love beans, just add some seasonings to them and they taste so good! Kidney, navy, black, and garbanzo beans are packed with fiber and protein. They provide high-quality fuel to keep you moving through your workout and all day.

Tomatoes—tomatoes are a great source of iron. Tomatoes are grouped with vegetables that help prevent certain types of cancer, heart disease and fatigue.

Garlic and Onions—these stinky things are rich in antioxidants this dynamic duo prevents injuries and keeps the heart in peak condition. Garlic lowers cholesterol, while the components in onions help the liver to detoxify waste products. Sautee your onions and add them to some of your foods for added flavor. Afterwards, pop a piece of ginger candy in you mouth to eliminate the bad breath!

Berries—antioxidant packed berries, like blueberries and cranberries, are loaded with vitamins C, E and carotenoids, which are good for the heart and help to prevent injuries and protect against cancer. These tiny fruits are filled with iron, which helps red blood cells carry oxygen and prevents fatigue.

Dried Fruits—dried figs and apricots pack a fiber punch, contain iron, and are convenient to carry and consume as a quick snack. Drink plenty of water to accommodate the extra fiber you intake.

Eggs—a great source of high quality protein, eggs are one of the few foods that contain vitamin D, along with a slew of vitamins and minerals, including iron for stamina, and all the essential amino acids. I enjoy egg white omelets, umm, umm good!

Fats—are essential for good health, brain development, and energy. The three major types of fatty acids include saturated, mostly found in dairy foods and fatty meats, polyunsaturated found in safflower, corn, sunflower oils, and certain fish and monounsaturated found in nuts, olive and canola oils. Not all fat is bad for you; the key is to exercise intake control. Choose small amounts of food with polyunsaturated or monounsaturated fatty acids to benefit from this essential energy source. The excessive fatty diet of many Americans is a major cause of obesity, cardiovascular disease, and high blood pressure. A healthy diet should include between 20 to no more than 35 percent of daily calories from total fat. A heart healthy diet should have less than 10 percent of total calories from saturated fat! The key is to select the right types and portion control!

Nuts—rich in protein provide important vitamins and minerals needed for muscle recovery and repair. For example, peanuts are a good source of monounsaturated fats and other nutrients, they reduce cardiovascular disease and in addition, peanuts have strong satiety properties, we feel full after eating peanuts.

Olive Oil—is fundamental to the Mediterranean diet, this delicious oil partners naturally with tomatoes, enhancing their antioxidant qualities. When you choose olive oil, you protect yourself against colon, breast, and skin cancer, as well as coronary heart disease, diabetes, and aging, while helping to reduce blood pressure levels. After all, a healthy heart is imperative for more energy!

I want you to be successful in your transition, so I have provided a meal plan for your first ten days. It features breakfast, lunch, two snacks and a dinner everyday! This meal plan incorporated with routine exercise helps to increase your body's metabolism. Thus, while you are sitting at your desk on a call, stuck in traffic or folding laundry your body should start to burn calories. Take some time to look it over and please make any substitutions needed to prevent allergic reactions.

10 Day Jump Start Meal Plan

Day 1—

BREAKFAST—Waffle with Cottage Cheese, Blueberries, and Turkey Bacon
- 1 multigrain waffle
- 1 cup low fat cottage cheese
- 1 cup fresh blueberries
- 1 slice low-fat turkey bacon

SNACK—Small (12 oz cup skim Cappuccino)

LUNCH—Tuna Salad
- 3 oz water packed tuna, drained
- 1 Tbsp. Capers
- 1 cup shredded romaine lettuce
- 1 cup raw spinach, chopped
- 1/3 cup onion, chopped
- 1 cooked egg white
- 2 tsp. mustard
- 1 Tbsp. Olive oil

Combine ingredients and serve.

SNACK—Celery and Peanut Butter
- 3 stalks of celery
- 1 Tbsp. Peanut butter

DINNER—Chicken and Snow Pea Stir-Fry on Brown Rice
- 4 oz. Skinless chicken breast, sliced
- ¼ cup cooked brown rice
- 1 cup snow peas
- ½ onion, chopped
- 2 Tbsp. Soy sauce

Stir Fry chicken, add vegetables. Cook until tender. Add soy sauce. Serve over brown rice.

Day 2—

BREAKFAST—Broccoli Omelet
- 3 egg whites and 1 whole egg, beaten together
- 1 cup broccoli

SNACK—Almonds and Grapes
- 1 cup grapes
- ¼ cup unsalted almonds

LUNCH—Turkey Sandwich
- 1 slice whole wheat bread
- 3 slices turkey
- 4 leaves romaine lettuce
- 1 tsp. Mustard
- 2 slices tomato
- 1 cup alfalfa sprouts

SNACK—Cottage Cheese and Paprika
- 1 cup nonfat cottage cheese
- 1 tsp. Paprika

DINNER—Salmon, Asparagus, and Salad
- 5 oz. Broiled or baked salmon filet
- 2 cups shredded romaine lettuce
- 1 cup chopped steamed asparagus
- 1 cup sliced cucumbers
- 1-½ Tbsp. Balsamic Vinaigrette

Day 3—

BREAKFAST—Tomato Omelet
- 4 egg whites and 1 whole egg, beaten together
- ½ tomato, chopped

SNACK—Raw Almonds and Dried Cranberries

10 raw almonds

2 Tbsp. Dried cranberries

LUNCH—Roast Beef Reuben and Salad
- 4 oz. Lean roast beef
- ¼ cup sauerkraut
- 1 Tbsp. Mustard
- 1 slice rye bread
- 1 cup shredded romaine lettuce
- 1 Tb. Balsamic Vinaigrette
- 1 dill pickle

Spread mustard on bread., layer roast beef and sauerkraut onto bread, then, serve with salad and pickle.

SNACK—Strawberry Yogurt Parfait
- 1 cup quartered strawberries
- 1 (6 oz) vanilla low-fat yogurt

DINNER—Chicken Burrito with Rice and Beans
- 4 oz. Skinless chicken breast
- 2 Tbsp. salsa
- 1 low-fat whole wheat tortilla
- ¼ cup canned pinto beans or black beans
- ¼ cup cooked brown rice

Arrange chicken and salsa on tortilla, then heat in oven or microwave. Toss rice and beans together.

Day 4—

BREAKFAST—Cottage Cheese and Raspberries
- 1 cup low fat cottage cheese
- 1/2 cup fresh raspberries

SNACK—Pear and Low-Fat Cheese
- 1 pear
- 4 1 oz. Slices low-fat cheddar or Colby cheese

LUNCH—Turkey and Avocado Sandwich or Wrap
- 3 1 oz. Slices turkey
- 1 slice whole wheat bread or whole wheat tortilla
- 4 leaves romaine lettuce
- 1 tsp. Mustard
- 2 slices tomato
- 1 oz. Raw avocado

SNACK—Celery and Peanut Butter
- 3 stalks of celery
- 1 Tbsp. Peanut butter

DINNER—Halibut, Broccoli, and Salad
- 3 oz. Baked or Broiled Halibut
- 1 cup steamed broccoli
- 2 cups shredded lettuce
- ½ oz. Vinegar
- 1 Tbsp. Olive Oil

Day 5—

BREAKFAST—Scrambled Eggs with Turkey
- 5 egg whites and 1 whole egg, scrambled
- 3 thin slices of deli turkey breast meat

SNACK—Yogurt and Almonds
- 1 (6 oz) vanilla low-fat yogurt
- ¼ cup chopped almonds

LUNCH—Chicken Pita
- 3 oz. Broiled skinless chicken breast, sliced
- 2 slices tomato
- 1 cup alfalfa sprouts
- 1 cup shredded lettuce
- 1-½ Tbsp. Fat free ranch dressing
- 1 low-fat whole wheat pita

SNACK—Peanut Butter Toast
- 1 slice whole wheat or multi-grain bread toasted
- 1 Tbsp. Peanut butter

DINNER—Steak, Brussels sprouts, and Salad
- 3 oz. Lean beefsteak or flank steak, broiled
- 1 cup Brussels sprouts
- 1 cup shredded lettuce
- 1 Tbsp. Balsamic Vinaigrette Dressing

Day 6—

BREAKFAST—Feta, Black Olive, and Tomato Omelet
- 5 egg whites and 1 whole egg, beaten together
- ½ cup black olives, chopped
- ½ oz. Feta cheese
- ¼ medium tomato, chopped

SNACK—Fruit and Cheese
- ½ apple or 1 cup red grapes
- 2 slices low-fat cheddar cheese

LUNCH—Turkey and Hummus Pita
- 3 slices lean turkey
- 1 small low-fat whole wheat pita
- 1 Tbsp. Hummus
- 4 lettuce leaves
- 2 slices tomato
- 1 tsp. mustard

SNACK—Whole grain crackers (such as Kashi) and Peanut Butter
- 5 whole grain crackers
- 1 Tbsp. Peanut butter

DINNER—Grilled Ahi Tuna Salad
- 4 oz. Raw, fresh tuna steak
- ¼ cup water chestnuts, chopped
- ½ oz. Sesame seeds
- 2 Tbsp. Lime soy vinaigrette*
- 1 oz. Soybeans
- ¼ cup papaya
- 2 cups arugula

Grill tuna for two to four minutes on each side then slice thinly. Arrange arugula on plate. Sprinkle soybeans and water chestnuts on top. Add papaya and tuna last. Garnish with sesame seeds and drizzle with lime soy vinaigrette.

*Combine ½ cup rice vinegar, ½ cup low sodium soy sauce, ½ cup fresh lime juice, 4 tsp. Dark sesame oil, 2 tsp. Lemon zest, 2 tsp. Fresh ginger, 4 cloves minced garlic.

Day 7—

    BREAKFAST—Breakfast Burrito
- 3 egg whites and 1 whole egg, scrambled together
- 1 small low-fat whole wheat or low-carb tortilla, warmed
- ¼ cup canned pinto or black beans
- 2 Tbsp. salsa

    SNACK—Small (12 oz cup skim Cappuccino)

    LUNCH—Chicken Salad
- 4 oz broiled, skinless chicken breast, chopped
- 1 cup shredded romaine lettuce
- 1/4 cup onion, chopped
- ½ cup cucumber
- ½ cup arugula
- 1 Tbsp. Balsamic Dressing

   Combine ingredients and serve.

    SNACK—Cottage Cheese and Tomatoes
- ½ cup low-fat cottage cheese
- 1 sliced tomato

    DINNER—Pork/Lamb Chop and Apple
- 4 oz. Lean boneless, broiled pork chop
- ½ apple

Day 8—

BREAKFAST—Cheese and Tomato Omelet
- 6 egg whites, beaten together
- ½ oz. Fat-free Parmesan cheese
- 1 medium tomato, chopped

SNACK—Almonds
- 20 almonds

LUNCH—Salmon and Salad
- 4 oz. Salmon
- ¼ cup onion, chopped
- ½ cup arugula
- 1 cup shredded romaine lettuce
- 1 Tbsp. Balsamic Vinaigrette

SNACK—Tropical Fruit Parfait
- 1 (6 oz.) vanilla low-fat yogurt
- 1 (4 oz.) cup pineapple chunks
- 2 Tbsp. Chopped walnuts

Top yogurt with pineapple chunks and chopped walnuts.

DINNER—Chicken with Peas and Carrots
- 4 oz. Skinless chicken breast, baked or broiled
- 1 cup peas and carrots

Day 9—

    BREAKFAST—Cottage Cheese and Raspberries
- 1 cup low fat cottage cheese
- 1/2 cup fresh raspberries

    SNACK—Celery and Peanut Butter
- 2 stalks celery
- 1 Tbsp. Peanut butter

    LUNCH—Chicken Curry
- 2 oz broiled skinless chicken breast, chopped
- ¼ cup cooked long-grain brown rice
- ½ cup raw cauliflower
- ¼ cup chickpeas
- ¼ clove garlic
- 1 oz. Tomato paste
- ¾ cup low-sodium chicken broth
- ½ Tbsp. Curry powder.

Simmer broth, then, add curry powder, tomato paste, and vegetables. Cover with lid, and cook until tender. Add chicken and heat through. Serve over brown rice.

    SNACK—Pear, Cheese, and Olives
- 1 medium sliced pear
- 1 low-fat string cheese
- 4 large black olives

    DINNER—Hawaiian Chicken Kebabs
- 3 oz. chicken breast, baked or broiled
- 3 strips yellow pepper
- ¼ cup pineapple
- ½ cup onion, chopped
- 1/2 cup cherry tomatoes
- ½ oz. Vinegar
- 1 Tbsp. Olive Oil

Thread chicken, pineapples, and vegetables onto skewers, drizzle with vinegar and oil, and cook on grill.

Day 10—

   BREAKFAST—Broccoli and Feta Omelet
*   5 egg whites and 1 whole egg, beaten together
*   1 cup raw broccoli, chopped
*   ½ oz. Feta cheese, crumbled

   SNACK—Celery and Peanut Butter
*   3 stalks celery
*   1 Tbsp. peanut butter

   LUNCH—Turkey Burger
*   3 oz cooked ground turkey
*   2 slices tomato
*   1 slice onion
*   1 Tbsp. ketchup
*   3 leaves romaine lettuce
*   1 cup alfalfa sprouts
*   1 tsp. mustard

   SNACK—Yogurt with Kiwi and Flaxseed
*   1 cup plain non-fat yogurt
*   1 kiwi, peeled and sliced
*   1 Tbsp. Flaxseeds (optional)

   DINNER—Chicken Pita
*   2 oz. Broiled chicken breast, sliced
*   ½ onion, chopped
*   ½ cup shredded low-fat Swiss cheese
*   ½ cup tomato sauce
*   1 small low-fat whole wheat pita

Heat tomato sauce, add onion, cover pan, and cook until tender. Place chicken in pita, pour sauce over and top with cheese.

The jump-start meals provided are 1100-1200 calories per day. I realize the change in intake may seem alarming, but as we discussed previously in this chapter, for weight loss it is necessary.

—Feel free to contact me at quantumquestonline.com for an extended personal nutrition plan-

Notice this is not a diet, it is a meal plan suggesting healthy meals and snacks as you begin your healthy lifestyle. I would never promote a diet, for one simple reason, they don't work!

Diets tell us exactly what and how much food to eat, regardless of our preferences and individual relationships with hunger and satiety. Dieting can help us lose weight, fat, muscle and water. Does that sound healthy to you? I don't think so, diets are so unnatural and unrealistic, that they can never become a lifestyle we can live with, let alone enjoy. Very few diets teach healthy low-fat shopping techniques, cooking, or dining-out strategies. Instead, many offer unrealistic recommendations and encourage health-threatening restrictions.

More importantly, diets don't teach us the safest, most effective ways to exercise; they don't teach us how to deal with our cravings or, how to attend to our feelings of hunger and fullness. Eventually, we become tired of the complexity, the hunger, the lack of flavor, the lack of flexibility, the lack of energy, and the feeling of deprivation. We quit our diets and the result is sometimes worse than the beginning. You know what I'm talking about, as soon as we quit, we gain more than what we started with! Every time we try a diet of deprivation, the weight becomes more and more difficult to lose. We become frustrated and discouraged and before we know it were eating more and exercising less, causing ourselves more frustration, disappointment and depression. Preoccupation with body shape, size, and weight creates an unhealthy lifestyle of emotional and physical deprivation.

Diets ultimately take control away from us. We are often caught up, in a "yo-yo" cycle that begins with low self-acceptance resulting in structured eating and living, because we lack trust in our body and are unwilling to listen and adhere to our body's signals of hunger and fullness. Instead, we depend on diet plans, measured portions, and a prescribed frequency for eating. As a result, many of us have lost the ability to eat in response to our physical needs; we experience feelings of deprivation, then binge, and finally terminate our "health" program. This in turn leads to guilt, defeat, weight gain, low self-esteem, and then we're back to the beginning of the yo-yo diet cycle. Rather than making us feel better about ourselves, diets set us up for failure and erode our self-esteem. The attitudes and practices acquired through years of dieting are likely to result in body weight and size obsession, low self-esteem, poor nutrition and excessive or inadequate exercise. Weight loss from following a rigid diet is usually temporary, because most diets are too drastic to maintain. When your diet fails to keep the weight off, you may say to yourself, "If only I didn't love food so much ... If I could just exercise more often ... If I just had more will power." The problem is not personal weakness or lack of will power. Only 5 percent of people who go on diets are successful.

Please understand that we are not failing diets; diets are failing us. The reason 95 percent of all traditional diets fail is simple. When you go on a low-calorie diet, your body thinks you are starving; it actually becomes more efficient at storing fat by slowing down your metabolism. When you stop this unrealistic eating plan, your metabolism is still slow and ineffi-cient that you gain the weight back even faster, even though you may still be eating less than you were before you went on the diet. In addition, low-calorie diets cause you to lose both muscle and fat in equal amounts. However, when you eventually gain back the weight, it is all fat and not muscle, causing your metabolism to slow down even more. Now you have extra weight, a less healthy body composition, and a less attractive phy-sique. The common theory is that, if you eat fewer calories than, you burn you will lose weight. However, when you eat fewer calories than your body needs to maintain its life-sustaining activities you're actually losing muscle in addition to fat. Your body breaks down its own muscles to provide the needed energy for survival. For long-term good health, you need to move away from low-calorie diets and focus on enjoyable physical activity and good nutrition. Exercising regularly and eating lean-supporting calories, protein, "good" carbohydrates and reducing fat-supporting calories will not only help you look and feel better, it will also significantly reduce your risk of disease.

Ditch the diet! Take the frustration, guilt, and deprivation out of weight management, and allow yourself to adopt gradual, realistic changes into your life that will make healthy eating and physical activity a permanent pleasure. You will soon discover what your body is capable of and begin to look, act, and feel your best.

"I am powerful."

Chapter 5: Maintaining the New Me

Tip*Consult your physician before beginning a vitamin and supplement regimen, to avoid complications with prescribed medication

Who needs vitamins? Everyone.
That was easy, but the real questions are what type, what brand, and how many?
Surprises, surprise, the answers to these questions are simple too, are you ready?
It depends on you!
Vitamins are potent compounds that perform many tasks in the body. They promote growth, reproduction and help maintain health and wellness of life overall. Vitamins constantly work to keep our nerves and skin healthy; they build bone, teeth, blood and heal wounds, among a list of other things.
They also help our bodies to work efficiently burning the calories we bring in through consumption.

According to the American Dietetic Association (ADA) and the American Medical Association (AMA), most healthy people meet their vitamin and mineral needs through a balanced diet. However, these same organizations say taking a multivitamin, under the guidance of a physician or dietician may be in order for the following groups of people:
(This is a shortened list it does not include all groups) Consult your physician for more information.

• People following low calorie diets

• People with certain diseases or those taking medications that interfere with appetite, absorption, or excretion of nutrients

• Strict vegetarians, whose diets may fall short of vitamin B12, Vitamin D, Calcium, iron, and zinc

• Women who are pregnant or breastfeeding, phases that bolster the need for nutrients, including iron

- Women with excessive menstrual bleeding, who may need iron supplements

- Anyone with lactose intolerance or who does not consume milk or other dairy products needs a source of calcium; those with an inadequate source of sunlight may require additional vitamin D

- Elderly people, with difficulty maintaining an adequate diet, chewing problems, or a reduced ability to absorb and metabolize certain nutrients

- People recovering from surgery, burn injuries, or other illnesses that increase nutrient needs

- People with heart disease or who are at risk for heart disease and consume diets inadequate in antioxidant nutrients (vitamins C and E) and B vitamins Ex: (vitamin B6, and vitamin B12)

- People with chronic diseases of the digestive tract or other conditions that lead to poor intake or deplete nutrient storage

- People with alcohol or other drug addictions are likely to have a shortage of vitamins and minerals in their diets.

If you decide to take a vitamin supplement, please keep the following points in mind while making your choice:

- Remember that price is not an indication of quality.

- Look for the product that meets high standards for manufacturing. Check the label to see if the product meets USP standards (manufacturing practices set forth by the U.S. Pharmacopeia, the organization that establishes drug standards. The organization's standards require that a supplement be able to disintegrate and dissolve thoroughly in the stomach within a certain period of time, thereby increasing the chances that the nutrients inside are absorbed and used by the body.

- Look for a bottle or package that has an expiration date. If the product does not show an expiration date, you will run the risk of buying a product that has been sitting on the shelf for a long period of time, losing its potency.

- Look for a supplement that contains both vitamins and minerals, with no more than 100 percent to 150 percent of the recommended Daily Values for each.

- Stay away from products containing extraneous substances such as PABA, hesperidins, inositol, and bee pollen, these substances have not been confirmed as essential dietary substances. These substances only add to the price of the supplement.

- Buy products sold in childproof bottles or packages if you have children around. Vitamins and minerals, especially iron, can be highly toxic to children.

- Be weary of taking multivitamins that contain herbs. Although herbal products are considered to be dietary supplements, the unregulated herbal industry today is a buyer-beware market. Source—FDA.gov (Food and Drug Administration)

Another way to maintain your healthy body is to exercise in the a.m. Morning exercise jump starts your metabolism, keeping it elevated for up to 24 hours! As a result, you burn more calories all day long. Not to mention the gratification of knowing you have done something positive and beneficial for your mental and physical health.

Exercise significantly increases mental activity allowing you to utilize that brainpower, instead of wasting it while snoozing. Once you have decided to make exercise a true priority, you will find that the world won't cease to turn if you get up 30 to 60 minutes earlier than usual. Especially since regular exercise usually means a higher quality of sleep, which in turn means you will probably require less sleep. (If getting up 30 to 60 minutes earlier each day seems too daunting, you can ease into it, starting with 10 to 20 minutes.) If you exercise every morning around the same time, your body will naturally regulate its endocrine system and circadian rhythms. As a result, your body will learn and follow your new schedule to a "t", your body will actually prepare itself to wake up and exercise before you even open your eyes! The body is truly a magnificent creation.

Fact: More than 90% of those who exercise consistently have a morning fitness routine. If you want to exercise on a regular basis, the odds are in your favor if you squeeze your workout into the a.m.

The feedback on a.m. routines has been very positive. The majority of my clients prefer the morning workout. They say there is an exhilarating feeling of accomplishment before the day even begins.

The beauty of a lifestyle change is that life does not stop. You in no way cease to live, you can experience all that life has to offer with an added bonus, a longer and healthier life. Here are 22 tips from the National Restaurant Association to guide you, while eating out without the guilty afterthoughts.

1. Order salad dressings and other sauces on the side, this way, you have control over how much or how little you add.

2. When ordering grilled fish or vegetables, ask for grilled food without butter, oil, or prepared "light," with little oil or butter.

3. When ordering pasta dishes look for tomato-based sauces, rather than cream-based sauces. Tomato-based sauces are much lower in fat and calories. In addition, the tomato sauce (or marinara sauce) can count as a vegetable!

4. Drink water, or unsweetened tea instead of regular soda or alcoholic beverages. This will reduce your caloric intake.

5. Share a dessert with a friend, half the dessert equals half the calories.

6. Share an appetizer. Same rule as above applies.

7. Soup can serve as an appetizer or entrée. When choosing a soup, keep in mind that cream-based soups are higher in fat and calories than other soups.

8. Order steamed vegetables as a side dish instead of starch.

9. Ask for salsa with a baked potato instead of sour cream, butter, cheese, or bacon. Salsa is very low in calories and a healthy alternative with a lot of spice.

10. Stop eating when you are full—listen to the cues your body gives you.

11. Order sandwiches with mustard rather than mayonnaise or "special sauce." Mustard adds flavor with virtually no calories.

12. Take half of your meal home. The second half can serve as a second meal! Don't feel obligated to stuff yourself.

13. To eat less order two appetizers or an appetizer and a salad as your meal.

14. If you have a choice of side dishes, opt for a baked potato or steamed vegetables rather than French fries. If choices are not listed, still ask your server to substitute vegetables or a baked potato in place of the French fries.

15. Look for items on the menu that are baked, grilled, dry-sautéed, broiled, poached, or steamed. These cooking techniques use less fat in the food preparation and are generally lower in calories.

16. The restaurant industry is one of hospitality and customer choice. Don't be afraid to ask for special low-calorie or low-fat preparation of a menu item.

17. Plain bread or yeast rolls are relatively low in fat and calories. It's the butter and oil you add that increases the fat and calories.

18. Choose entrees with fruits and vegetables as key ingredients. Enjoy the flavors they offer. Fruits and vegetables are a good source of dietary fiber, vitamins and minerals.

19. Choose foods made with whole grains like whole-wheat bread and dishes made with brown rice.

20. Herbs add a unique flavor to any dish! Try foods flavored with fresh herbs rather than fats such as oil and butter.

21. If you have a craving for a dessert, opt for something low fat like sorbet, fresh berries or fruit.

22. Remember not to deprive yourself of the foods you love. All foods can fit into a well-balanced diet.

Always be Aware of Portion Size

"All things in moderation", is a school of thought that believes this theory is all it takes to achieve and maintain a healthy weight. With that in mind, let's take a look at some simple portion control techniques that will surprise you—they're very easy to do and what a difference they make!

Meet Yourself Halfway

You *can* lose weight and still eat your favorite foods! Just decrease your portion sizes by half. For example, if you usually eat a whole deli or sub sandwich at lunch, just eat half, and supplement your meal with raw veggies on the side and finish with fresh fruit. Then wait to see if you're still hungry. If you pause after eating the first half and allow yourself a few minutes to feel satiated, you just may find that you are too full to eat the other half anyway! DO NOT eat until you are full!

Never Be Ashamed to Ask for a Doggie Bag

Restaurant portions are unbelievable — nearly twice the size they were 15 years ago. When dining out, ask the waiter for a take out container as soon as he brings the food. Go ahead and put some of your food in the box as soon as it arrives. You can always take some back out while at the restaurant if you're still hungry, but chances are you won't want to. Heat the leftovers the following day for lunch.

Downsize that Dinner

Many restaurants offer lunch size portions of their dishes, which are smaller than their full-size dinner entrees. Don't be afraid to ask if you can purchase the lunch size entree at dinnertime. If you are feeling like a kid at heart, ask to order from the children's menu! If you tell your server you are watching your weight, they usually allow it. Practicing this tip will save your waistline some inches and your wallet some bucks!

No Mega-Super-Biggie Size Anything

Fast food portions are *over*-sized, so there is no need to add insult to injury by *super*-sizing. No matter how much money they claim you save just say no. In fact, steering clear of "meal deals" altogether is very wise. You are much better off ordering a chicken sandwich or burger and a side salad. Another tip is to order a kids meal. Kid's meals contain what *used* to be normal sized portions for adults (Before there were "value" meals or combos).

Good Portions Come in Small Packages

If you find your will power is overpowered by a full bag of popcorn sitting in the pantry, don't buy the large bags and select the popcorn without added salt and butter to lower your caloric intake. Don't buy the 12-bag assortment box if you think you will be tempted to finish the entire box in one sitting! Instead, buy the individual lunch size bags one at a time. Another tip is to divide the popcorn into single serving snack bags as soon as you get home.

Size Up Your Servings

How many (Your favorite snack here_____) are in a serving? Check the box you may be surprised at how many servings you are actually consuming. Measure your favorite snack to learn what a controlled portion looks like, then, you will be able to "eyeball" it for future reference, knowing exactly how much is too much.

Buffets be Gone!

My boys love buffets, I on the other hand avoid them! It is nearly impossible to practice portion control in an "all-you-can-eat" situation. If you have ever left a buffet feeling sick, just think about that the next time you are tempted to gorge.

Learn and Remember the Standards

Three ounces of meat is the size of a deck of cards or an audio tape; 1 oz. of meat is the size of a matchbook; 1 cup of potatoes, rice or pasta looks like a tennis ball.

You Can Do This!

Everyone tells us to stay motivated. Our friends, our co-workers, our relatives say to keep going, don't quit. Sometimes, though, you ask, "Why? Why try my hardest when it ends in disappointment? Because it's going to be different this time! Because you can't accomplish anything, if you give up. Disappointments and failures happen to everyone. (Remember my intro ladies!) The difference between those who reach their goals and those who don't is motivation. If you are motivated, you'll keep going. If you keep going, you will reach your goal. Use the following points to keep the fire burning inside you.

Build Confidence

How did you feel the first time you walked the stairs at work/home without losing your breath? The more you accomplish the more you will believe in yourself.

Bring Sexy Back, with an Outfit from Your Past (not too far in the past!)

It's been hanging up in your closet for two years now, just waiting to be worn for a night out on the town. All it takes is for you to go that extra mile and stay on track. Before you know it, those two years will be ancient history.

Enjoy your Days, Nights and Weekends

Have you ever felt like the week was taking forever? It feels like Friday, but it's only Tuesday! This happens when you are not working towards anything. When you have a goal in mind you'll want to cook that healthy dinner or go to the gym. The week will not only seem faster, but more enjoyable.

Give Yourself a Purpose

Sometimes we need a reason to get out of bed. If your health and wellbeing aren't two great reasons, then I don't know what is. Eat a healthy breakfast to jump start your day, go for your morning jog, or walk to grab the newspaper.

Do it for your children and your grand children

The healthier you are, the longer you'll be around to watch your kids grow and spoil your grandchildren. Consider this another bonus.

Learn the Power of Momentum

It's a scientific fact—something in motion stays in motion. Momentum builds quickly and can lead to great results. Suddenly, you're not only working for the goal, but also competing to keep your winning streak alive. More reason to fight to reach your goals. Besides you only live once, go for it!

The "Wow" Effect

Picture this: You run into someone from high school, and his or her eyes light up. They gasp, "Wow, you look great!" By sticking with your goals, this can happen. Watch the "wows" add up!

Spread the Spark

When family and friends see how hard you're working; they'll wonder how they can reach their goals. Guess who they are going to look to for help? By staying motivated, you'll not only help yourself, but others too.

Keep Gaining Experience

The more you do, the more you will learn and understand. You will discover which tactics work best for you. It's like your favorite perfume; it doesn't smell good on everybody.

Stay Healthy Naturally!

(Always obtain physician clearance prior to beginning any exercise program.)

Take it Slow!

Never exercise without warming up to avoid injury.

Work It Out!

Set 30 to 45 minutes aside at least 3 times per week. As your workout progresses increase the time. (Try a circuit- use 2 to 3 different cardio machines.)

Mix it Up!

The body adapts after 4 to 6 weeks so, add variety to avoid weight loss and fitness plateaus.

a.   Change the mode of exercise

b.   Change the speed and intensity (incorporate inclines and/or intervals)

c.   Try a Group Exercise Class

d.   Weight and Strength Training increases energy levels and increases bone density

e.   Cardiovascular Training helps your cardio-respiratory system function more effectively

EAT Realistically!

Avoid drastic changes in your eating habits. The goal is to build healthy eating habits you can live with.

Rotate!

Rotate all foods every 24 hours; for example, if you eat chicken on Monday avoid it on Tuesday.

Trade It!

Many food alternatives high in protein or low in calories can be substituted for food containing less desirable characteristics.

*TIPS:

a.   Grate cheese do not slice it.

b.   Try fat-free pretzels instead of chips.

c.   Eat whole grains avoid white starches.

It's Okay to Crave!

It is human nature to crave things; the key is to monitor your portion size. Relax; it is okay to include a serving or two into your meal plan.

In closing, success means nothing if we are not healthy enough to enjoy it. I urge you to make your health a priority. If you need encouragement, refer back to the promises you made to yourself while reading this book. I have shared my personal and professional experiences with you, so I hope you consider me a friend who truly has your health and happiness in mind.

The most important thing I learned throughout this process is to have faith. Before the layoff, I liked to plan everything; but I learned not to place so much energy into planning but to preserve it, so that I can roll with the opportunities that come my way. Through it all, I came to realize that whatever I desired to do; I could achieve it if I set my mind to it. You can too. This book's premise is to inspire you to go after your dreams despite the ("It's") that stand in your way. Stay focused, stay motivated and if no one supports you, I support you in your quest for a fit and healthy life.

"Don't Let "IT" Get You!"

JOY

978-0-595-46709-9
0-595-46709-1